# C-Sharp Minor:
## My Mother's Seventeen-Year Journey through Dementia

# *C-SHARP MINOR:*

## MY MOTHER'S SEVENTEEN-YEAR
## JOURNEY THROUGH DEMENTIA

DEBORAH P. HALL

XULON ELITE

Xulon Press Elite
2301 Lucien Way #415
Maitland, FL 32751
407.339.4217
www.xulonpress.com

Exulon
LITE

Unless otherwise indicated, Scripture quotations taken
from the King James Version (KJV) – *public domain*.

Scripture quotations taken from the New American
Standard Bible (NASB). Copyright © 1960, 1962,
1963, 1968, 1971, 1972, 1973, 1975, 1977, 1995 by
The Lockman Foundation. Used by permission. All
rights reserved.

Printed in the United States of America.

ISBN-13: 978-1-54564-407-2

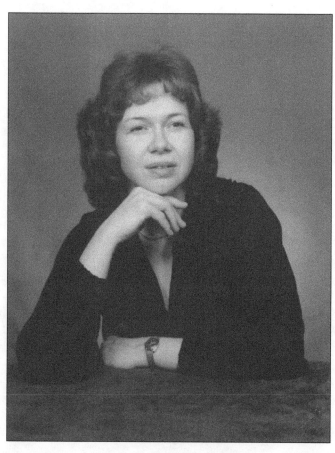

**Photo Credit: Olan Mills**

*For Mom*
*"I thank my God in all my remembrance of you."*
*Philippians 1:3 (NASB)*

# *Table of Contents*

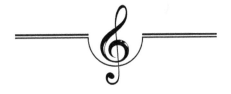

# Prologue

# *C-Sharp Minor*

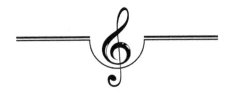

*P*relude in C-Sharp Minor. The piece will always be an invitation to memory for me, drawing me back decades to one unforgettable recital when Mom bit off more than she really could chew and, as usual, still managed somehow to swallow.

Mom's piano playing, like the rest of her, was powered by sheer determination. Her true musical talent lay in singing, her passionate, pure tones coming straight from the heart, but she enjoyed piano just for herself. That didn't mean she took it casually. Even Mom's recreation always had purpose, goals, and challenges. She was incapable of taking it easy on anything, least of all on herself.

She acquired the first piano that was her own after we moved up to the same town as her parents following a house fire. She bought it on payments soon after we transitioned into our newly built house, and when we kids started piano lessons, she as an adult signed up as well.

The piano lessons of her childhood had come from her mother. Mom hadn't particularly applied herself in those early years, as their styles differed significantly. Grandmother's strict "everything three times perfect before you go on" system had crashed head on into Mom's free-spirited individualism. Mom had ample self-discipline, but all her life, she rebelled against rigidly defined systems.

Later she confessed to me that she regretted her lack of application in those early lessons. Personality differences had interfered with learning music, and she mourned the lost opportunity, for she *loved* music. From childhood clear through her teen years, she always saved up her allowance for records and books. Now and then, Grandmother would try to interest her in clothes or other pretty things, and Mom would look at her in pure bewilderment and reply, "What would I want clothes for? I already have some."

Thus Mom, in her midthirties when she bought her piano, started lessons right along with us. Because of those earlier aborted efforts and her lifetime of intense involvement in singing, she wasn't beginning from step one as we children were. She already read music well, and she could play in a careful manner. Still, that wasn't enough. She wanted to *play*, realizing that she would never match her beloved records, but wanting to narrow the gap. She threw herself into lessons with vigor, trying to make up for lost years, practicing late at night.

Her favorite piano solo all her life had been Rachmaninoff's *Prelude in C-Sharp Minor*. As she started lessons, she chose that piece as her goal. Mrs. Burnett, the old lady who taught a host of kids (and a few adults) piano in the neighboring town, did point out that the *Prelude* is very difficult and that it would take a while to master that advanced work.

Mom characteristically tried to whittle down the definition of "a while." All her life, if faced with a prediction that it would take her this much time to accomplish something, she responded by throwing full effort into trying to beat the estimate. She drilled that piece night after night, forcing her fingers to learn it, and if she lacked Rachmaninoff's genius of expression, she certainly wasn't short on willpower.

Mrs. Burnett gave yearly recitals of her students, and when a recital down at the local church rolled around, Mom insisted on going with the *Prelude*. She could play it by then, adequately if not spectacularly, and she wouldn't accept anything else for her recital piece. The day of the recital came, and the students played in increasing order of difficulty, so Mom and Rachmaninoff shared the last slot on the program.

The *Prelude in C-Sharp Minor* begins famously with three emphatic chords: *Dum! Dum! Dum!* Rachmaninoff is said to have been inspired by bells, and you can almost see them tolling high above in tall towers. After that, there comes a brief pause, then an answering, softer echo. Those three chords and the gentler reply form one of the most recognizable openings in classical piano literature.

Mom sat down at the piano, adjusted the bench back for longer legs than the children's, took a deep breath, and began, playing by memory as Mrs. Burnett insisted all her students do at recital, even the beginners. The chords rang out firmly through the old stone church.

*Dum! Dum! CLANG!*

She missed the last one, hopelessly missed it, leaving no doubt in the mind of even the least musical member of the audience that this was an error. Mom came to a dead stop, frustration sweeping clear through her posture, up to her face, and then erupting in one emphatic, fortissimo exclamation.

"FISH FEATHERS!"

The audience broke up laughing, and Mom jumped and looked over, as if only then remembering she was in public. Grim determination knocked frustration to the mat, and she squared her shoulders and turned back to the keyboard. Once again, she started, this time daring either the keys or her fingers not to cooperate. *Dum! Dum! Dum!* And off into the remainder of the *Prelude*. The rest of the piece went well, but it somehow sounded not so much like Rachmaninoff as like Mom. At the end, the audience applauded, and Mom stood up and descended the stairs with a satisfied air, even if still tinged with the memory of the error. She had achieved her goal.

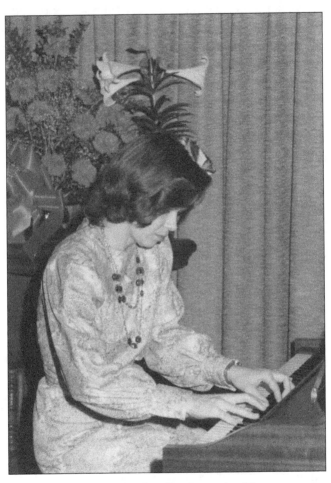

**Mom playing Rachmaninoff**

\*\*\*

We started down the concrete staircase at the edge of the parking garage, and I watched Mom walk beside me. Her movements held a certain tentativeness about them now. They weren't yet slowed beyond normal for most people but definitely were diminished from her lifelong full-speed-ahead approach to anything. It was not a limp, and she didn't have any trouble with the stairs. Her footfalls were even, just not as sure. On questioning over the last months, she had assured me that nothing was hurting except for the occasional weather-related ache from an old leg injury years ago. Mom was vehemently anti-doctor and getting even more so, but on subtle checks, nothing seemed wrong with her eyes. ("Oh, look at that cat across the road. Do you see her, Mom?" "Yes, what a pretty calico!")

No, the physical slowing was tied to the mental, as if life itself were off balance, her mind in danger of falling. It was early autumn of 2007, and Mom was sick. Her memory was in slow but steady decline at that point.

At least she had Erdenheim. I took comfort in the thought that night. Erdenheim, my beloved farm, which she loved almost as much, the land that both of us called the most peaceful place on earth. When she had reached the point of forgetfulness that I was doubting her ability to live independently a few years before, I had bought a used mobile home and set it up in my backyard. Mom contentedly lived in her own place only seventy-five feet away from my house. At the farm, my youngest brother, who shared her trailer, and I could keep a closer eye on her as she walked progressively more slowly into mental twilight. Fortunately, she had occupied only the latest in a string of rental houses before the move, and she had been glad to come to the farm, not seeing it as a loss of her place.

She never outright mentioned the mental issues, but she knew. Now and then, in unguarded and oriented moments, I could see the flash of fear in her eyes. But she was happy there, and I hoped she would be able to live out her life at Erdenheim with me.

Tonight, we were going to the symphony to hear Rachmaninoff's *Second Piano Concerto*. As the *Prelude in C-Sharp Minor* had been her favorite piano solo, so the concerto was her favorite orchestral piano piece. Formerly, we were regulars at the symphony, but we hadn't gone for a few years. However, when I heard a radio commercial for this concert and mentioned to the family that I was planning to go, my middle brother sent us money for two tickets. I thought this quite likely would be her last opportunity to hear the great work live, for Mom, as the confusion advanced, was getting uneasy in large crowds of strangers, unable to process all the multisided stimulation. Indeed, as we entered the building after half a block's walk from the garage, she edged slightly closer to me, like a child afraid of losing the parent. Our roles had been reversed.

By the time we found our seats and sat down, I was starting to wonder whether this had been a good idea after all. Perhaps already it was too late. The large hall bustled with activity, the cacophony of hundreds of conversations competing with the orchestra's jumble of last-minute practice of the individual instruments. Mom was unsettled, not quite panicked but heading there.

I tried desperately for distraction. "What do you think we should plant at Erdenheim in the spring?" I asked. She loved flowers and plants and had landscaped every place she'd ever lived, even though only one of those houses of her life had been owned and not rented.

She seized the topic like a mental lifeline. "We could use a few smaller bushes around my trailer to go with the pink flowering almond and the potentilla. Maybe a euonymus." Her words were flawless, even on the more difficult terms. Up until nearly the final year of her life, Mom's speech would remain intact, and up until the last four or five years, she would be able to fool people in short conversation, defending her decline as fiercely and as futilely as the soldiers had the Alamo.

Finally, to my relief, the lights dimmed, and the concert master and then the conductor and guest pianist stepped out on the stage. The sea of sound in the room dropped instantly into almost imperceptible gentle waves of anticipation.

Then the music started. The pianist opened the work alone, a series of fifteen chords in statement and reply, building toward the first theme and the entrance of the orchestra. Again, and even more so than in the *Prelude*, it evoked bells tolling, but here there was no dramatic pause in the music—only relentless gathering momentum.

Mom straightened up, and her eyes focused. *Her* eyes, her old eyes, the uncertainty of her new world dropping away. The music carried her back to whole days. I sat there half watching the excellent pianist and appreciating the work, half watching her. She never noticed; she was mesmerized as she had been from her very first encounter with classical music at age three.

Her parents actually had thought she was sick because, while with them on a pastoral visit, she had sat rapt, perfectly still beside a record player that was pouring forth Beethoven's *Third Symphony*. Mom was almost never perfectly still, but from that first experience, even as a very active toddler, music was the exception. When fully listening to music, not performing it herself but listening, she was respectfully and completely focused, her spirit at reverent attention for every single note. All else fell away, and those moments were defined only in sound.

So it was on this night of the concert, as once again the music captivated her. For me, the feelings of the night were as varied and intense as the piece. Gratitude. Sorrow. Fear that I wouldn't be able to be enough, to give enough on the road ahead. Mourning. Joy. Pure lyrical beauty.

Rachmaninoff has few equals for music you can *feel* when under stress, the full gamut of emotions, all wrapped up in one composition. That is precisely why Mom loved the *Prelude* so much. She told me several times over the years, "It has such feeling. So much passion. Even in the quiet parts, it's solemn and pensive, and then there's that middle. So much going on there, busy, hectic, scrambling, sometimes agitated even, but with all that, there's still beauty that pops through. It's like life. And at the end, there's a resolution and that lift."

Ah, yes, a resolution. I hated, as did she, works ending still in conflict, the struggle without the resolution. Give us the struggle, the depth, the range, but there *must* be a resolution.

Tonight, thinking of the road ahead, I looked toward the ending. I knew the ending, and yes, there was resolution, there was clear harmony waiting ahead. The score was written down, and while I didn't know all the piece, I knew that in the end, ultimately, there would be healing and freedom. It was the middle, those yet-undefined-to-me pages, from which I shrank.

*Focus on the moment,* I reminded myself. Don't add the worries of tomorrow in advance when today has quite enough to deal with already. Tonight was a special gift to her. Appreciate it, live it, give thanks.

And tomorrow? And next year?

I did not know, but I knew that I wasn't responsible for knowing. God knew, the same God who gave us the gift of music, who we are told sings over us. *Lord,* I prayed, *help me let that be enough.*

Rachmaninoff ended, and Mom turned to me, still at that moment in her old self, and enthused, "That was *wonderful!*"

"Yes," I agreed.

*Thank you, Lord, for this night. Thank you for the music.*

Even in the hardest times, there was still music.

# 1.

## *Early Days*

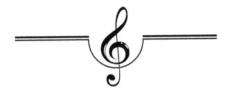

F rom the beginning, Mom refused to conform precisely to expectations. She was born at seven
months' gestation on Easter Sunday. Granddaddy,
a preacher, really had had other plans and responsibilities already on his agenda for Easter Sunday.
Furthermore, Mom was a girl. She had been expected
to be a boy, and all name-considering sessions between
Grandmother and Granddaddy had relied upon that
prediction. Thus, for a girl, they had nothing ready
and were left scrambling at the hospital.

That oversight often amused Mom in later years
as characteristic. Granddaddy, while he had a heart
as large as the Pacific Ocean, wasn't the most prac-
tical-minded person in terms of application, and
Grandmother, who was intensely practical, had
trouble conceiving any action on her part that devi-
ated from "how it should be done." She probably had
nightmares about failing to meet expectations, and she
was always readier to forgive lapses on the part of
anyone else before her own. With everyone expecting

a boy, she assumed automatically that it was therefore her assigned duty to have a boy.

Then along came Mom. She was premature and undersized but tough as nails, putting up a good fight for herself. The hospital was overcrowded, plenty of wartime babies arriving, and there wasn't an incubator available. Mom won the battle on her own. The staff was soon ready to discharge her, but they refused to let her leave without Mom having a name. Grandmother and Granddaddy finally came up with Paulette, but that sole candidate exhausted their imagination, and they never could arrive at a middle name. Thus, Mom had no middle name throughout her life, a fact over which she got into a few fights with official forms.

She was a very active, bright, strong-willed child. She wasn't often outright defiant, but she had a strong scientific bent even from an early age and wanted to experience things and explore her world. She went straight at life full speed. She often in later years appreciated the home she was born into and said that given her personality, had she not had rock-solid morals and loving-but-firm discipline with boundaries surrounding her, she might well have gotten into trouble (of the legal, criminal variety) when she became older.

Granddaddy was the primary disciplinarian, though both would act if needed. Nor did it always take the form of spanking, which was reserved for high offenses. Mom remembered that when Granddaddy had to correct her, he was incredibly painstaking to make sure that she fully understood her sin and how it could have been handled otherwise. She would be sitting there outwardly attentive during the parental lecture but wishing he would just go on and get to the consequences. Nothing was ever done in anger, but there were definite expectations of behavior, and she was required to meet them. That simply was never up for debate in that house.

Always precocious, she was talking in full sentences by the time she was one. Grandmother and Granddaddy often took her along on pastoral visits, and in her early years, she was much more often around adults than other children.

It was on one of those visits that she had her landmark first encounter with classical music at age three. Grandmother and Granddaddy both liked music, but neither of them was into classical. Grandmother always played the radio while she did housework, listening to the popular music of the day, and was also frequently the pianist at the various churches they served and would practice at home. Thus both at home and at church, Mom was exposed to hymns and liked them. Granddaddy enjoyed country and bluegrass, which Grandmother definitely did not. Mom well remembered Grandmother saying to him, "Oh! That whoo-whoo-whoo music! Turn it off!"

At the church member's house that memorable day sat an old Victrola, something Grandmother and Granddaddy lacked, though Mom was given a record player by Granddaddy a few years later. The church member had just put on Beethoven's *Third Symphony* as they arrived, and Mom instantly gravitated to the record.

A fireworks display on the Fourth of July wouldn't have been as riveting. She sat absolutely still, mesmerized by sound. When Grandmother asked worriedly if she was feeling sick, she shushed her impatiently.

She didn't want to talk; she wanted to listen to the music. The one time she started getting upset in that visit was when the record ended, and the homeowner made her day by telling her, "I can just turn it over, sweetie." Even on the ride home, she remained silent, and when Grandmother asked her what she was doing, she answered, "I'm listening to the music again in my head." For Mom with classical, it was love at first sound.

Granddaddy talked to her at length about church. He emphasized how she must be quiet and never disrupt a service. Someone might be dealing with the Lord, and a distraction might break that solemn moment. Her parents did give her plenty of times to run and play actively, but there were appropriate places as well as inappropriate ones for that. Church was always to be respected. That led to another fond (in retrospect) memory that Mom often told.

Sitting in a church service one toddler day, she had long since lost interest in the sermon. There was no separate children's church then, and she was wondering how much longer this would go on. Daydreaming had its limits, and she started shifting around, first quietly, then more vigorously. She didn't even realize what she was doing until Grandmother bent to pick up her purse from the floor, and Mom knew that she was about to be taken out. Being removed from a church service was sure to have further repercussions at home.

Trying to think of a quick way of escape, her mind seized on the seemingly perfect answer. Granddaddy was up at the front preaching. Granddaddy would *never* disrupt the flow of a church service himself. Never. She couldn't imagine it. As Grandmother reached out to take her arm, Mom scampered into the aisle, ran down it, climbed onto the platform, and hid behind Granddaddy and the pulpit. Granddaddy, to her absolute amazement, stopped at once in mid sermon. He stepped back, looked down at her, and simply said, "Come get her, Ivy Dean."

Grandmother hurried down the aisle to collect her stray daughter, and Mom was indeed taken out of church, only she got to be marched the entire length of the sanctuary in front of God and everybody. And yes, there definitely were further repercussions at home.

There was also, however, an alternative activity presented after that for future services where she was bored. By that point Mom had already learned to read. Their house was not a house of books, aside from the religious commentaries in Granddaddy's study, but he always read the newspaper beginning to end every morning. Mom would climb into his lap and ask what he was doing, and he started reading it aloud to her, then following the text with his finger. He never pushed her to read in any way, but Mom from the beginning had to learn, had to know. Education was as appealing to her personality as play even at that age, and once told the paper contained information that he was reading, she wouldn't let it alone. She quickly grasped the concepts of letters and words, and that newspaper became her Dick and Jane. I've wondered if getting a full dose of current events each morning from toddlerhood on impacted Mom's later love for and, in her early decline, near obsession with politics and what was going on in the world.

By age three, she was reading fluently. After her church escapade, Granddaddy told her that if she was getting bored in a service, she could simply grab the hymnal out of the rack in front of her and read it. Quietly reading was an acceptable alternative, and Mom loved to read and would never get restless doing that. So she read that hymnal cover to cover, over and over. This was, I'm sure, the root of her encyclopedic knowledge of every verse to *everything*.

This did lead once to a dispute with the children's teacher in Sunday School. The preschool class of assorted-aged young kids had to sing "the stupidest," in Mom's opinion, songs. They were silly, they lacked musicality, and she thought the repertoire could definitely be improved. So, Mom at age three asked the teacher if they could sing something else. The teacher asked what she would like to sing instead, and Mom replied, "The good hymns, the ones that aren't silly songs. Things like 'Guide Me, O Thou Great Jehovah.'"

The teacher stared at her for a moment, taken aback, then patiently explained, "Paulette, the children don't know that one."

Mom didn't consider that an obstacle at all. "Well, it's right there in the hymnal. They could read it." The answer that the other children could not read left Mom flabbergasted. How could *anybody* not read and not be actively working day and night to correct that deficiency?

The family moved from southern Arkansas, where she was born, to Kentucky when Mom was a toddler, and Granddaddy attended seminary in Louisville while still pastoring. When Mom was about four, he took her on a visit, not a pastoral visit but just a field trip for her, to a horse farm owned by an acquaintance. At the end, they were standing in a pasture next to a horse that had been haltered for petting. The man lifted Mom up and set her on the horse's back while he continued chatting with Granddaddy.

Mom sat there sorting out all the aspects of this experience, her first up-close encounter with horses, and then she did the thing that, according to Grandmother's radio dramas and the few movies she'd seen, was correct behavior for when you mounted a horse. She kicked him as hard as she could and yelled, "Yah!"

The horse spooked and bolted, lead rope pulled loose and flying. For Mom, there was no fear at all. She had asked him to run, and he was obediently running. She remembered clearly the ground rushing by, the wind in her face, and the smooth action of the powerful galloping legs pounding beneath her. She held on to the mane, but she was laughing, enjoying every stride. The radio dramas and the movies had it right; this was *fun*.

The ride of her young life didn't last long. The owner quickly grabbed another horse, jumped up himself, and set off in fast pursuit. He caught them, seized the rope, and pulled her horse back down to a walk. Mom remembered him starting to reassure her, only to be interrupted. "Can we do that again?" It wasn't until they returned to Granddaddy, who was white as a sheet, that it occurred to her that anything might be wrong with that whole action sequence.

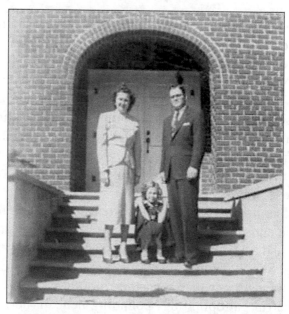

**Mom with her parents on the church steps.**

The family's first television arrived in the house when Mom was six. Granddaddy promptly sat down to watch it before she was allowed, and he carefully viewed all shows available, which at that time was a short list, and sorted out which were six-year-old appropriate. He then presented to her the shows she was allowed to watch and told her that she was not to have the set on during any others. Mom tried to push that a time or two, more in curiosity than defiance, but Grandmother, even working in the next room, always kept her ears attuned. Mom would try to leave the TV on after her show finished, but she never got more than two words into the opening theme song of the first forbidden show before Grandmother would be saying, "Paulette," in *that* tone.

It was about this time that, once she was going to school, Mom asked Granddaddy for some terminology lessons. She told him that she had noticed that other children in school referred to black people by different names than he did, and she wondered what she should call them. Granddaddy told her, "If you are talking to them, you call them ma'am or sir, just the same as you would any other adult. There's no difference. In general, you call them black, and you do not use those words the other children use." She replied, "Yes, sir," and that issue was settled.

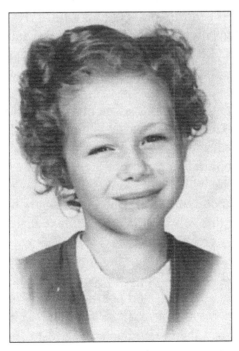

**The young Mom could have doubled for Shirley Temple.**

The family moved around often, especially after Granddaddy graduated from seminary. Everywhere she lived, Mom had a few good friends but wasn't particularly close to most of her classmates. The best part of school was, of course, the library. She read voraciously, and librarians soon stopped trying to steer her toward books intended for her age level.

It was at age nine that she prayed a prayer very typical of Mom's personality, but one that she later admitted she wished to take back. Mom had accepted Jesus at age six, and she often prayed in bed at night after she was supposed to be asleep, extending the supervised bedtime prayers into a full private conversation. This night, she prayed, "Lord, I want to experience it all. All the emotions of life. I want the lows as well as the highs. I want to know despair as well as joy. Let me see *all* of it."

Her tenth birthday was memorable for unpleasant reasons. Her gift was a new bicycle, and she was thrilled. Granddaddy provided her with a detailed parental reminder of appropriate riding rules and road safety along with it, but she was occupied watching the bicycle, smooth and sleek. She already knew how to ride them, but this was the first big-girl bike that was hers.

Finally freed to ride, she took off down the street and then stopped riding straight. Mom started doing swirls and loop-de-loops, enjoying the motion. Other kids were watching, and she began showing off her birthday prize and her skill in handling it, changing to one hand and then to no hands. She lost control, went flying, and hit the pavement *hard*. Later, she told me how she saw stars at the impact and how everything was tilted and somewhat blurry after that.

Undoubtedly, she had a concussion. It was several days before her vision stabilized and the headache left. Nobody noticed that at the time, though, because she never mentioned it in all the concern over her badly broken left collarbone. She saw the X-rays herself. The bone was dangling like a swing seat when one rope has broken. The old GP in the town said that it might require surgery, and Granddaddy was about to face dutifully the cost of this when the GP suggested trying an alternative first. He wanted Mom to spend the next week in bed with her arms straight out shoulders to elbows, then raised from elbows to hands. No guarantees, but he thought that *might* pull the bone piece back into alignment. If there was no improvement by the follow-up X-ray, he would have no choice left but to refer her to a specialist for surgery.

So Mom spent that week in bed, hands up. It had been emphasized that she was never to be allowed to put her arms down, not once. Others fed her, and when she went to the bathroom, Grandmother supported her hands, holding them up until she got back in bed. This enforced absolute bedrest also helped the head injury she hadn't thought to mention to anyone, and by the time of her return visit to the GP, she could see straight again. The follow-up X-ray showed that the collarbone had indeed pulled back roughly into alignment. Everyone breathed a prayer of thanks, and Mom returned home still on guarded activity.

Meanwhile, of course, there was the issue of punishment. Granddaddy knew from the report of the other kids that she had been cutting up and breaking many of the safe-riding rules he had just given her, and there must be consequences. He decided that her punishment would be that she was grounded from riding her new birthday bicycle for six weeks. It would be parked there on the porch, and she would have to walk by it going in and out the door every time, but it would remain off limits. However, since she was out of commission for six weeks first with the collarbone, he decided that time didn't count. She wouldn't have been able to ride anyway, so that was healing time and could not serve simultaneously as disciplinary time. Her six weeks of grounding would not start until she was fit to be riding the bike again.

Therefore, for a total of twelve weeks, first with the collarbone and then serving out her sentence, she had to look at that bicycle, walk by it multiple times a day, and never take it out. Many times throughout that period, Granddaddy made her tell him again what she had done wrong, how she should have known better, and why this was her own fault. Once her time was served and she was released onto the streets again, she was the safest bike rider imaginable. "When Granddaddy gave you consequences for something," she said later, "he did a good job of it. You definitely remembered it." She never admitted the head injury until years later, but the topic of possible effects from it would come up again in the course of her final illness.

Mom's sister, Vicki, arrived when Mom was ten, and a whole new dimension entered the household. Vicki, a strong will herself, though quite different in personality from Mom, could never understand why the acceptable activities for the girls weren't the same. Thus Vicki, ten years younger, resented Mom for being allowed to go to school, go out with friends to activities, and even, in her midteens, go on dates. Once in a while, Vicki got to go along just to shut her up; Mom remembered outings where she was fifteen, and Vicki, sitting with a satisfied smirk in the back seat, was five.

Those teen years also marked Mom's first cat. Mom had had a dog or two when she was a child, none staying with them long for various reasons, but she had always been especially drawn to cats. Grandmother, however, did not want a cat around. So Mom lived reluctantly catless up until Vicki got a Chihuahua. Vicki had severe allergies as a child, and the dog was prescribed by a doctor who knew that the breed had an oil in their coats that was good for allergies. Thus Vicki, by doctor's orders, was assigned to sleep with a Chihuahua.

Mom at once appealed to the court of Granddaddy that this was not fair. If Vicki was allowed a special personal pet, even if for medicinal reasons, Mom should be treated likewise, because there were also nonmedical pet benefits that Vicki would be receiving that Mom always had been denied. Granddaddy, who was nothing if not fair, considered this argument and concluded that she was right. That was the start of Vicki's lifetime love affair with Chihuahuas and Mom's with cats.

Her first of countless cats was named Su Ling, a black cat but with shading in the sunlight. Vicki, of course, was unable to leave Mom's cat alone and even took a notion to dress her in doll clothes. Vicki had inherited Grandmother's interest in clothes that Mom lacked, and she loved playing dress up, whether with herself or other objects.

Again and again, Vicki would seize Su Ling and start to dress her, and the cat would give one growl. Vicki would ignore this and plow straight on with what she was doing, and the cat would give a second, louder growl. Vicki once again would pay no attention, and Su

Ling would then switch to a stronger language. When Vicki ran crying and bleeding to Grandmother and Granddaddy, the parental court ruled again in favor of the cat. "She warned you twice," Granddaddy would say. "We aren't going to punish the cat; you had a chance to stop. It was your own fault." A few days later, the same scene would be played out yet again. Nobody in this family ever lacked in determination.

It was in her junior high and high school years that Mom became more interested in writing. She was on the committee to edit the yearbook several times, and she enjoyed playing with words herself. Along the way, she wrote her one really good poem, a memory of seasons in Kentucky in her early childhood.

Writing, however, was soon replaced by other time-consuming interests. One of her regrets later in life was giving up the efforts at writing and turning down the full-ride scholarship she was offered to Ouachita Baptist University, choosing instead to start a family. She was always careful to explain to me that she never regretted *us*. Mom loved her children with everything in her. But she regretted turning down the scholarship. She wondered, in a road-not-taken sort of way, what that other life might have held and whether she might have actually accomplished anything eventually of her writing. Perhaps she could have had both that and family if she had chosen differently.

Nevertheless, she had some satisfaction looking back at her literary phase. "I did it once. There was 'Kentucky.' I wrote something that really clicked once, so I did get to experience what that was like. I just wish that it had truly been able to be published."

That much, Mom, I can give you.

## Kentucky

*The world is young, 'though the year be old*
*In Kentucky.*
*The lilies smell on each spring-found knell*
*Of all the essence of hope and love;*
*The rain-drenched moss sweetly doth emboss*
*The heav'n-swept tree as a foot-worn glove;*
*And spring leads summer to autumn's gold*
*In Kentucky.*

*A hidden stream in a hushed wood*
*In Kentucky*
*Strokes time-worn roots while its gentle flutes*
*Pour melody forth to waiting trees.*
*When autumn turns all the green-clad ferns*
*To brown, and leaves overlay the leas,*
*Then gusts of wind play where flowers stood*
*In Kentucky.*

*When winter roars in the white-blest land*
*In Kentucky,*
*Or calmly shakes by the icy lakes*
*The boughs of fairyland color caught*
*In crystal cold in their morning mold*
*Of stillness, all life's joy is wrought*
*In living, confident in the hand*
*Of Kentucky.*

# 2.

# *Slaying Lizards*

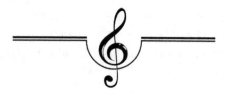

M om met Dad in California, where he was just finishing his service in the navy, and they were married with Granddaddy performing the ceremony. My oldest brother was born a little over a year later, and shortly thereafter, the new family moved back to Georgia, Dad's birthplace, to be near his family.

"We always moved not long after I had a baby," Mom commented once, remembering dealing with the packing and upheaval along with the newborn. This was the longest move of her life, clear across the continent, but she was grateful for the change because it was then that she got to live close to Dad's mother for several years. Grandma was one of those simple but wise people who was ever full of good advice, and Mom always had the highest respect for her. Even later, after the divorce and move to Missouri, they talked at times on the phone.

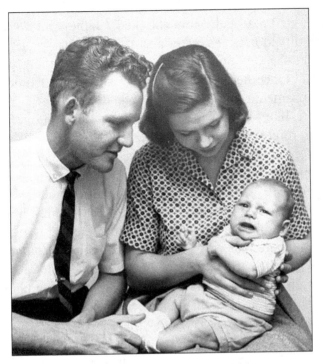

**Dad, Mom, and Michael.**

Brother Michael was followed three years later by James, the one Mom said was probably partial payback for her own strong will as a child. James' exploits included the time he discovered one toddler day that the holly bush at the corner of the house reached up above the roof. Nobody had expected him to be anywhere near climbing trees yet, but when Mom's back was turned for a moment dealing with Michael over something, James swarmed up that bush with impressive speed, arriving on the roof. When she turned around and spotted the missing child, he was trotting at full toddler tilt across the roof, interested in seeing where this shingled road led. Mom shrieked, "James! Sit *down*!" He turned back, gave her a surprised look, wondering what she was upset about, and responded cheerfully, "Hi!" Once he was retrieved, the shrub was trimmed that same day.

I, like Mom, was expected to be a boy and in fact was referred to among the family as Thomas Wiley before my birth, but Mom privately already had a girl's name in reserve. She had prayed for a daughter—not specifically during that pregnancy but in general, years ago, before marriage. She always had wanted many children, but she had prayed that at some point among them, there would be at least one daughter. She named me Deborah after the judge of Israel and Paulette after herself, and when talking to her parents on the phone not long after, she told them, "See, I didn't have trouble finding something that goes with Paulette."

The three of us children were within five years of each other and played together, but James was the ringleader and experimentalist. Michael was the responsible one, trying his best to keep activities from leading into trouble, and I was quiet. One of James' science experiments that I remember came the day he heard them announce on the radio that "it's hot enough to fry an egg on the sidewalk." We lived in Atlanta just then, and James felt compelled to test this theory. He took an entire dozen eggs from the refrigerator and tried them out in full shade, partial shade, full sunlight, and varying stages in between. The experiment was successful, and every time I hear that phrase since, I remember that in Atlanta in the summer, in anything except full shade, you can indeed fry an egg on the sidewalk.

Another childhood adventure came in what we referred to as the four-story house. This was actually a split level, with a double staircase at the end of a long dining room that went both ways to partial upper and lower floors. There was a full basement beneath all of that. I loved that house, for it was marvelous to create stories in. In its heyday, it had been impressive, though it was now rather the worse for wear and was a rental property. Next to it reigned a magnificent oak tree, and as tall as the house was, the first branch of that oak was taller still. Mom specifically noted that fact with relief, as James loose on that far-taller and multilevel roof would have been a nightmare.

The staircase at the end of that dining room had a full two-story drop at its tallest point from the upper level to the lower, and one day Mom found James tying me up into a laundry basket over my squirming efforts to break free. She asked him what he thought he was doing, and he replied that the Sunday School lesson the last Sunday had covered Paul being lowered over the city wall in a basket to escape those who wanted to kill him. James planned to recreate this scene at that stair-case, lowering me over the rail at the top in the laundry basket. Mom objected vehemently to this plan, and James innocently replied, "But I learned this in church!"

Another great memory of that house is the music. Mom always sang, no matter where she lived, but at that house, she would sit in the upper hallway at night after putting us to bed, all of the bedroom doors open, and softly sing us to sleep. The peaceful river of sound flowing through the doorway from the hall would carry me off into pleasant dreams.

Music was an eternal presence in her life and in ours while we lived with her. She sang while driving, while doing housework, and, of course, in church. James, copying her, actually could sing "Jesus Loves Me" on the correct tune before he could even speak the words. He would belt out at full volume, "La la la la, la la la! La la la la, la la la!" She had fond memories of people being startled by this.

James and I were the two who inherited her love of singing the most. Michael never really got into singing, though he was better than he thought he was, but he played the trumpet in the band in school. Later on, my youngest brother, Daniel, was also a decent singer but, more than any of us, was talented on instruments. He played piano and also violin and was a member of the youth symphony.

Mom sang plenty of hymns, of course, but she also had working songs, "get-er-dun" songs, and others for all occasions. One she loved to sing as encouragement to us when we were small children was "High Hopes," about the ant who thinks he can move a rubber tree plant. She also had mistake songs, some of which I think she made up herself. Those were sung more to herself than us. She always was hardest on herself for mistakes, having that much of Grandmother in her. To this day, I can remember her annoyed rendition of an apparent original, "If you don't do it right, you get to do it over." She sang "Sixteen Tons" sometimes while doing housework. Whenever she would trip over something or perform some other feat of incoordination, she would launch into the chorus of "Grace That Is Greater Than All Our Sin," giving it an ironic inflection on the first two words as she addressed those to herself: "Grace, grace."[1]

Then there was the "something on top of the car" song, which I know she made up. That was inspired by her driving off with a coffee cup on top of the car one morning and having it fall off at a curve and shatter. From then on, whenever Mom, with hands overfull as usual, would set something on top of the car while juggling burdens and opening doors, she would start singing, "There's (coffee/Coke/a sack/whatever) on top of the car!" She would sing it forte while stowing the rest of her packages, and she was not allowed to stop until she had retrieved the temporarily parked item.

She did this in parking lots at stores as readily as in her own driveway, and many passersby looked curiously at Mom busily unloading her shopping cart and singing away. Mom, of course, didn't care a whit if people looked at her or not. She wouldn't go out of her way to appear odd just for oddness' sake, but provided she had a logical reason for her actions, and she rarely didn't, the opinion of the general public on its strangeness quotient was irrelevant.

She also wasn't above modifying songs now and then. She had never been a morning person. In fact, her family nickname of Polly was not a shortening of Paulette but itself came from a song. Granddaddy was an enthusiastic, if not overly talented, singer himself, and he used to sing to her to wake her up in the mornings. One of his favorites for this purpose was "Polly Wolly Doodle All Day," because he said she wanted to doodle all day in bed. She gradually became known in the house as Polly Wolly, which compressed over time to simply Polly.

The dislike of mornings continued all her life, and she sometimes trudged dutifully about the house on especially early days singing "Morning Has Broken" but changing the words and inserting her own second phrase: "Someone please fix it."

Mom and Dad divorced after twelve years of marriage. One thing that we kids appreciated was that through the remaining several years of our growing up, they always cooperated on us. We weren't made into pawns in a parental chess match as happens with some broken homes. Mom stayed at that point in Georgia. She had been for the most part a stay-at-home mom through the years of her marriage, but she now enrolled in a medical assistant course and entered her long career in doctors' offices. She was valedictorian of her class. She also bought the first car that ever had been truly hers. This was a bright red Volkswagen Bug that she named Leonardo da Vinci "because he's so versatile." Leonardo was to remain with the family for many, many years.

Mom never lacked for imagination, and now, driving alone to work for the first time in her life, entering Atlanta each morning from the suburbs, she created a game to pass the time. She would choose a historical figure from a previous era, such as George Washington or Queen Victoria, and she would explain the sights and the city to them, trying to frame it into their own context in the description. I am absolutely convinced that, had she gone on with it, she could have easily been a writer, most likely in science fiction or fantasy; she loved both genres.

About a year after the divorce came an event that had a profound impact on the family both then and later and would resurrect itself in the years of her illness. Mom and the three of us kids were living in Snellville, Georgia, in a rental house. (Daniel came from a later marriage and, as Mom often phrased it, "had not discovered America yet.")

The house's wiring was as old as it was, and one night, it caught on fire. This was in the middle of winter, as much winter as you got in Georgia, and it was cold that night. It was cold enough that Michael, who had the back bedroom, really an extension on the back of the house, slept instead in the living room next to the old standing gas heater. The fire started in his unoccupied bedroom, climbed the back wall, and got into the roof. By the time he woke up to get a drink and walked into the kitchen, he could see the flames flickering in the back of the house and reflecting through the windows from the ground outside.

He woke up Mom. We three children were her priority, of course, but after we were safely out and the fire department was called, she tried to grab a few things and throw them out the door onto the front yard. Giving it up as hopeless, she ran on out to join us. I will never forget standing out there at the edge of the street in our pajamas, cold to our backs, blazing heat in front, and watching our house burn down. The fire department came, but it was already so far gone that there was no saving it.

Mom had a good friend named Carmen who lived not far away. Carmen, herself a single mother of three children, took us into her home that night, and we lived there for the next several weeks. Most of our possessions were destroyed, and Dad took us clothes shopping the next day. I remember being embarrassed to be in the store in my pajamas, but it was all we had. After we bought clothes, we changed in the parking lot one at a time while lying down in the back of Dad's car.

We picked through the fire debris, and a few things were salvaged. Some pictures made it, scorched around the edges but still visible. James was annoyed that his GI Joe submarine had melted, while Michael mourned his silver dollar collection. This had contained over thirty silver dollars and had been in his bedroom, which burned the longest. The coins were now reduced to a silver lump. He threw it away in disgust, though I've wondered since if it still would have been worth something. A watering can that we children had given Mom for Christmas was also melted, which seemed to my young mind especially unfair. We had saved our allowances to give her that.

But several books made it, again with some singeing and smoke damage but still readable. Mom noted, "At every bookcase, something heavy had fallen across it and protected it." Remarkably, all of our Bibles made it and were far less damaged than the other books. I still have my Bible from that period. The cover is smoked slightly on one side, but the interior pages are bright white, pristine.

We had lost almost everything, but we still had our lives. Living with Carmen was rather packed with six kids, two adults, a few cats, and a dog in a not-too-large house, but it had its fun moments, too. One Saturday, we went to Stone Mountain. Leonardo had a Stone Mountain season pass, which applied to the vehicle, not to an individual. Carmen's much-larger station wagon did not. So to save admission, we piled into the Bug for the day's outing—six kids, two adults, and a dog.

Grandmother and Granddaddy at this point offered to help Mom get resettled, reestablished in a house, and help her with the kids. Thus it was that we moved to Missouri, where her parents had relocated from California years before. The neighborhood people donated enough after the fire that Mom had to get a U-Haul for the trip, with Leonardo attached behind and serving as a rolling cat carrier.

Once we moved to Aurora, we lived with Mom's parents for a while until our house was built. A new housing development was going up just one street over, and Mom signed on one of them early enough that we got to choose a few details in construction. I remember going over after school and inspecting the house each day, watching it be created. James, of course, wanted to help the crew.

When that house was finished, Mom was able to really indulge her love for plants and landscaping for the first time in her life. Even at rental houses, she always planted some things, but the Aurora house would be the one yard that she actually owned. I still remember her diagram on paper as she showed me what would go where. An orchard. A garden. A rose garden. All sorts of flower beds. All of it was planned most carefully with an eye to what the full-grown product would look like. She reveled in it, and that yard was one of the great joys of her life.

I was never as good at growing things as she was, but she let me help her tend them and weed the beds. Some of those plants I even called up from memory and put in at Erdenheim years later just because she had once gotten joy from them, but there was one point, literally, of disagreement between us in that Aurora yard. I called it the Wicked Thorn Tree, though the official title was Washington Hawthorne. It stood at the back corner of the yard with its impressive thorns, and it seemed to delight in reaching out to grab me at any opportunity. Mom told me that it just didn't like me and was much gentler with her.

Mom threw herself full speed into church activities, and she also became very involved at this stage, the latter half of the 1970s, with the singles ministry. The whole concept of having classes and outreach especially for singles was just getting established in the church, and she was working at the state level in the organization of this. I recall her many times heading off in Leonardo for a weekend conference at Windermere or Tan-Tar-A. She always got a kick out of packing Leonardo for a trip, enjoying the fact that the trunk was in the front. Mom appreciated things done not quite as expected.

It was also in the late 1970s that she started attending night school at a university in Springfield. She selected psychology as her major, being an incurable people watcher. It would take her over a decade to complete her bachelor's degree, although her second marriage certainly slowed down progress during that time, but Mom as ever doggedly stuck to it. Quit simply wasn't in her vocabulary.

Mom took determination to new heights. Nothing that she set her heart on ever received less than 150% effort, and now, juggling family, job, school, and church, she did her best at all of them. There is a TV animated special that is an adaptation of Rudyard Kipling's story "Rikki Tikki Tavi." In it, the mongoose travels so quickly from one place to another that often his back end is still around the last corner while his front paws are already on the other side of the room, and it takes a few seconds for the whole animal to catch up. That mongoose reminded me of Mom: full speed ahead, sometimes with the back paws scrambling a little bit in it all but always going somewhere. She laughed at this description and agreed that it was apt.

She had a very compassionate heart, and anyone truly in need had not only her sympathy but anything she could do to help. There were multiple times when someone else lived with the family temporarily, not just relatives but friends needing a landing pad for one reason or another for a while. Many times Mom paid forward Carmen's taking us in the night of the fire.

On the other hand, her quickness did make her impatient and volatile at times. Laziness was intolerable to her, and anyone she perceived as committing that sin rapidly lost all sympathy. She often said, "Our family has faults, but laziness is not one of them."

With businesses, she had much less tolerance than with people. Let a business once annoy Mom, and she could boycott it for decades. She even wrote steaming "angry consumer letters," as she called them, pointing out the faults of said company. Life's general difficulties were similarly irritating to her. Whatever patience she had was applied to people; companies or impersonal obstacles got none. Those were ever handled as a campaign, charging at them with iron determination to overcome.

It was in high school that I coined a phrase about her based on this tendency: slaying lizards. I told her, "Mom, slaying dragons is a noble occupation, but you don't need to slay lizards. They aren't worth the full effort and ceremony." She thought that was hilarious—she always could laugh at herself—but she went right on through life slaying lizards wherever they appeared.

The house in Aurora was always full of books and cats. Mom read voraciously, and as we kids grew, she worked very hard to provide reading matter that would interest us. I was easy; just make it about animals, especially horses. James enjoyed the science fiction and science fact that she herself did. I remember a large, well-thumbed book that he loved called *Mysteries of the Unexplained*, which was a compilation of strange occurrences like planes disappearing into the Bermuda Triangle. Michael, Mom discovered, appreciated the *Guinness Book of World Records*, and once she learned that, we always had the latest edition of it.

There was one well-remembered day in my childhood when Mom proved the high value she set on books. I was in sixth grade, and we had received the latest Scholastic book flyer a week or so before. I marked my choices and presented it to Mom for payment, but she was out of checks and waiting for a new order. She set it aside and said she'd give it to me later to turn in. However, a cat vet emergency occurred over the next few days, and both Mom and I forgot all about it.

I didn't realize until arriving at school that morning that this was the deadline for the book order. Mourning the missed books, I nevertheless decided that this was my deserved punishment for having forgotten about it. I should have reminded her. Therefore, I would take my sentence like a soldier and not mention it. I even planned to find the order later among her paperwork and remove it so she wouldn't feel guilty herself.

In the middle of these thoughts, there came a knock on the classroom door, and there stood Mom at the school in late morning, throwing her schedule totally awry, with the book order form and a check in hand. She smiled at me and handed it over. This was the one and only time I can ever remember Mom bailing out one of us on some forgotten item we didn't take to school; her usual attitude was tough luck, guess you'll remember it next time. But books were *important* in our household.

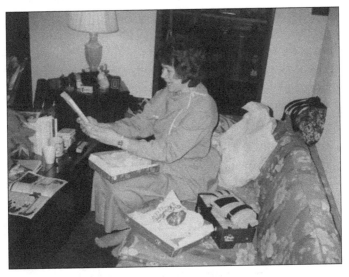

**The joy of a new book.**

Music continued to be central to our lives. She encouraged us in the church's children's and then youth choir, the piano lessons, and in band in school, but she also had an admirable flexibility, trying to fit to our individual tastes. I played clarinet for a while in band, but it never really was a source of joy, not like the singing. When I asked her for permission to quit, she let me. After she got her own piano, I asked her around age eight if I could practice at home alone instead of under Grandmother's eye at her house in the afternoons because Grandmother's three-times-perfect insistence was driving me nuts. Mom agreed, and my lessons didn't suffer for it. She always said that we had to try the band and the piano, but after a good trial, if we didn't want to continue, she wouldn't force us.

Band created another fond memory of Mom. Michael and James both continued on up into the marching band stages, Michael on trumpet and later James on trombone. The band would perform at half-time at the local football games, and Mom definitely wanted to be there for her sons to see and hear them. On the other hand, she hated sports. All her life, from her own school days on, she hated sports. For her, the halftime band performance was the whole point of the evening, not the game sandwiching it. She first tried dropping off the band member earlier and returning for halftime. It was difficult to predict exactly when that would come, and also, the traffic and parking lots were already at full jam before that, so after she was late a few times, Mom came up with a new plan.

She simply took a book or a crochet project. Mom would sit in the stands working on an afghan or immersed in a chapter, oblivious to the cheers and reactions of the football-watching crowd around her. When they all started to get up and head out to the restrooms or concessions, she would come to herself, realizing that halftime had arrived. Putting away the book or craft, she would watch the band with full, rapt attention.

Once they had finished, she would dive again into her own world and sit there through the rest of the game until she could collect her son afterward.

Grandmother, once she found this out, was absolutely horrified. "You can't *do* that!" she protested. "What will people think?" Mom's shrug made it perfectly clear how much it bothered her what people would think.

I was eleven years old when Mom managed to swing riding lessons. I was the only one in the family passionate about horses, but she always encouraged that once she saw it in me. Financial reality was an aspect of life, however, and riding lessons cost money. I wasn't shielded from that. As a child, I began helping her with balancing her checkbook each month, a task she hated and often fell behind on. I've always loved to organize things; cleaning my room was never an issue, and I even helped out in cleaning those of siblings. Weeding flower beds wasn't a chore but a straightening, an ordering of the world of those little plants, and I enjoyed it.

Similarly, balancing the checkbook, tracking down the occasional lost cent, was enjoyable to me, and once I discovered that fact, she let me do it from then on. She would supervise those sessions, but she really did dislike the job herself, as the occasional lost cent was distinctly unimpressed at her lectures to it. I was the one who loved to chase down any discrepancy, turning it into a numerical scavenger hunt; Mom merely got annoyed.

With the checkbook, therefore, I saw the figures monthly from about age eight on. I knew what there was and wasn't money for. It made the reality of riding lessons when it came that much more special, because

I knew she had worked hard to have that extra and had even sacrificed other things.

The day we went out to the stable for the first time to arrange lessons wound up being memorable for unexpected reasons. Mom admitted later that she had nightmares about it. That day also would form a baseline for me of "Mom with kid in medical crisis" that I could compare to a few events many years later, measuring her decline.

We went to the stable on a Sunday afternoon. Two days before, on Friday, James and I both had gone to the large medical clinic where Mom worked, taking the opportunity for some minor procedures as there was no school that day due to teachers' conference. We saw the same general surgeon. James had a few warts burned off his hands. I had a plantar wart on the bottom of my left foot that was becoming increasingly troublesome to walk on, and the doctor burned that off as well. He applied medicine and dressings for both of us, gave post-op instructions, and the appointment was over in twenty minutes.

I followed all instructions, but by Sunday, I knew something was wrong. The pain in that foot was steadily increasing, and that morning, I had trouble bearing weight at all. I also felt generally shaky and ill. But we were going to the stables that afternoon to arrange riding lessons, something I'd dreamed of for years, something I wasn't about to postpone for anything short of death now that it was here. I didn't tell anyone how I was feeling, and I made myself walk normally on that foot throughout church that morning and then in the tour of the stable that afternoon.

Once the first lesson was safely scheduled for the next weekend and we left, I asked Mom to pull over on the dirt road before we'd even gone half a mile. "I think something's wrong with this foot," I admitted. She stripped off shoe and sock, and there were red streaks heading up the leg. It hadn't looked that bad that morning, though I had had no doubt it was going wrong in some way.

Instead of turning right at the highway for the forty-five-minute journey to home, Mom turned left for the should-have-been-twenty-minute journey to the city to the ER. It took her less than twenty minutes. Yes, a Volkswagen Bug can do eighty. She was definitely worried and not trying to hide it, but she was focused and anything but scrambled. Again, I would remember that years later. She was smoothly but speedily efficient.

She lectured me thoroughly later that week on exactly what I'd done wrong. "You don't pull a stunt too often, but when you do, it's a good one." I meekly apologized for trying to conceal a septic foot and asked if we could still take the first scheduled lesson the next Saturday. She didn't have the heart to cancel it but said I had to be thoroughly un-striped and with normal temperature first. I was.

James, of course, had promptly disregarded all his post-procedure instructions. He went to his part-time job at the bowling alley the day after wart removal and put his hands in the industrial-strength cleaning solution that they used to clean the bowling machines. Mom had to roll her eyes after the dust had all settled. "James ignores every instruction, does everything wrong, and is perfectly fine. Deborah follows things to the letter and winds up at the hospital. It figures."

Mom always tried to listen to her children and was glad to hear us out, but there was no question who was in charge of the household. She used to say, "This house is a democracy, but my vote counts four." With three kids at that point, this stacked any vote in her favor. Another well-remembered saying was, "We'll have peace if I have to enforce it with war."

Her ample imagination extended to methods of punishment. She didn't mind using corporal punishment, but it was always reserved for truly serious offenses. For times when she just wanted to make a point but which didn't deserve a spanking, she had a few other methods. One favorite that she used when appropriate was Bible verse sentences. For instance, a sibling disagreement that went beyond the usual routine give-and-take and got serious was worth 500 from each involved party of, "Be ye kind one to another, tender hearted, forgiving one another even as God for Christ's sake hath forgiven you."[2] Chronic failure to clean a room might be worth 300 of, "Let all things be done decently and in order."[3]

The strictest sentence of sentences I ever knew her to hand out came during the short interval when my stepbrother, son of her second husband, was living with us. He left the hamster cage open one night, which in that house of cats was a death sentence. (He still protests his innocence and says that it was the cats who figured out the latch, though he had been careless with the cage on prior occasions.) Mom demanded 1500 rounds of, "A righteous man regardeth the life of his beast, but the tender mercies of the wicked are cruel,"[4] and she did put a tight deadline on that assignment.

In January 1983, Mom met her second husband. This relationship only lasted a couple of years and was in the end a disaster, though my little brother Daniel was very much planned and wanted. Gary was a type I'd never run into before, nor had Mom: charming, slick, the best liar I have ever met in my life. He was a con artist, plain and simple, and before long, the house and Mom's prized yard were sold, and the money was used by him, not her. He came across very well on first impression, and most people who knew him liked him for about the first six months. At that point, the more observant began to notice the picture forming as they spent more time around him. Many verified details on him came to light through a PI report a few years later that Mom ordered for ammunition during a custody battle. Mom had to learn the hard way, but we agreed afterward that Shakespeare summed him up perfectly: "One may smile and smile and be a villain."[5]

Michael and James both in turn had moved up to live with Dad during part of their high school years, so I was the one mainly around during that marriage. Gary set off my radar in a way that I couldn't explain, and at thirteen, I was too young to trust that inner voice and hoped for Mom's sake that I just was imagining things and uncertain about change. She was so obviously happy, at least at first. He knew to the max how to play someone. Like any con, he sensed that I wasn't quite sure of him, and he responded with a bribe: he was the one who gave me my first horse. The gift didn't work as intended; I loved the horse but still felt a little uneasy about him.

During the marriage, Gary's son, who had been living with his mother, came to stay with us for a while.

Mom's impact on him was monumental in that short time, and I was touched that years later, after her death, he took a couple-of-hour drive to attend her funeral. She was different from any of the adults he'd encountered in his life to that point. He especially remembered her quietly living out her faith and her matching his interests to reading material and getting him involved in books, something he'd never enjoyed before knowing her.

My brother Daniel was born in 1984. Mom had quit her medical clinic job at the end of the pregnancy, and keeping up the family tradition, we moved shortly after Daniel's birth. The Aurora house had been sold, and we relocated to the very small country town where Gary had an auto parts store with an apartment overhead. This town and that small upper apartment on the square were the catalysts for one of my all-time favorite Mom memories.

The square was bare. Painfully bare. There were a couple of trees, and that was it. Mom, the landscaper, the lover of flowers, was offended at this lack of beauty outside her window, and she offered to landscape the square at her expense and maintain it. The town powers that be turned her down because flowers and such were "too much bother."

Mom, thus officially thwarted, retreated to the apartment to look at that bare square and scheme. Then she ordered several bulbs. The town was so small that they practically rolled up the sidewalk at 10:00 p.m. during the week, everything quiet, and for several nights, Mom dressed in dark clothes and crept out at midnight armed with a hand spade. She planted bulbs, carefully arranging the beds, of course. I thought this was hilarious and asked if I could join in the party, so she let me come with her the last two nights. The next spring, she watched carefully, but the flowers weren't mowed down, and the square for at least the time she was there had its beds. Of course, they knew who had done it, but nothing was ever said.

Classic Mom. It ranks right up there for me with the fish feathers recital. The world needed flowers, and Mom was going to see that it got flowers. She would ask permission first, but with permission or not, the world was going to get flowers anyway.

Eventually, Gary's true character came to light, and the divorce was filed. Mom and Daniel and I moved then to an apartment in Springfield. That marriage shook Mom up badly. She had misjudged Gary completely, and she often admitted that. One thing that I loved about Mom; she owned up to mistakes. She was far from perfect, but I cannot count the number of times over the years that she said to me, "I was wrong. I blew it." After that divorce, she said that Gary proved that she was too naive and impulsive in some areas. She even asked me, into upper teen years at this point, to remind her of that fact if she ever started to get involved with another man.

We were so close, the two of us. So close. We always had been. I have read with wonder of the supposed phase where kids want to talk to or spend time with anyone else rather than their parent, but for me, it never came. Prior to her more advanced illness, there was not a single day of my life where she wouldn't have been my first choice for a human confidante. I could talk to her about anything, absolutely anything, and that feeling was mutual. Of course, she appropriately reserved some topics on her part until I was older, but even before that, she always shared with me her own dreams, her worries, her regrets, and her passions to some extent. We could talk about important issues facing us, or simply about flowers or animals, or not talk at all for hours, and it never grew old. We were truly friends.

We also read to each other, exchanging snippets back and forth, as we both loved wordcraft and poetry. Her favorite poem was by Theodore Tilton and was about a king who had a signet ring engraved with the saying, "Even this shall pass away."[6] That was his counsel, right there where he could see it easily, for any situation that came up. The poem starts, "Once in Persia reigned a king," and it goes on through assorted highlights of life, including triumphs, low points, pain, fame, and finally death, each stanza ending with, "Even this shall pass away."

Decades later, on the day that she left Erdenheim for the final time, when I was taking her to the nursing home, she started quoting that poem as we pulled out. "Once in Persia reigned..." There she hung, losing a poem that she had known by heart, that she had often quoted. The words wouldn't come. She kept trying. "Da da dum da dum da dum." Finally, the last repeated line came back to her. "Even this shall pass away." I had to fight back tears as I drove out of the driveway, taking her away.

In the year that I graduated high school, Granddaddy gave me as a graduation present two tickets to the Kentucky Derby. Mom and I made the trip cover four days, one to drive there, one to look around Lexington and Louisville, one at the Derby, one to drive home. Mom was as excited about this trip as I was, appreciating my own passion for horses and full of memories of her childhood years in Kentucky. We stayed at the KOA Kampground for budget reasons, and the night before the Derby, we had a conversation that would often come back to haunt me in future years. It was after dark, and the camp lantern had been extinguished. We lay there in the tent, each in a sleeping bag, too keyed up for the next day to sleep, chatting like girlfriends at a slumber party.

"What are you most afraid of?" she asked me.

I considered for a few moments. "Failing to meet a responsibility," I replied.

I could hear her smile in her tone. "You've got a lot of Grandmother in you."

"That's your doing," I pointed out. "We're related."

"Yes, I guess I am responsible for that."

"What are you most afraid of?" I asked her, curious.

She didn't have to pause for thought at all. The answer was immediate and decisive. "Losing control of my mind."

# 3.

# *Partners*

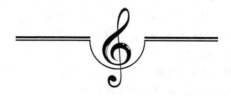

At the end of the summer after the Derby trip, I went off to college. Mom bought a new vehicle the week before she took me up, the second brand-new one of her lifetime. Leonardo, her first totally new car, had been passed on to James by this point, and our family car was an old Fairmont station wagon named Stumbler. Mom and I shared Stumbler, and in a reversal of the usual drill, I took Mom to work every morning rather than her taking me to school. I would have the car through the day and pick her up that evening. Stumbler was well past his prime and truly merited his name, and we had borrowed Granddaddy's vehicle for the Derby trip, but as the summer wore on, it was clear that Mom either had a choice of repair bills or car payment monthly. She chose the car payment.

Mom decided on a truck. "I've always wanted a truck," she said. "Not a great big ego truck, but a little versatile truck." She took me along with her car shopping, and she was as excited that day as a kid the night before Christmas. Mom's enthusiasm was one of her most memorable traits; she always threw herself into life at the fullest, and she allowed us children to see her passions and her excitement at the things she enjoyed. Buying that truck, giving herself a long-wanted treat as well as mere transportation, was fun for her. Still, she was deliberate, asking questions and looking at several choices. The first dealership was too pushy in her opinion, and she walked out, displaying her usual practice with businesses of "one strike and you're out." The salesman at the second car lot listened more respectfully and met with her approval.

She narrowed the selection down to two Ford Rangers and got stuck there momentarily, so she asked me to pick one of them. I did, and she bought that truck, but as we were leaving, she asked the reason behind my selection. It was simple. I had noticed that the official term for the color on one of them was chestnut, which, of course, reminded me of horses. She smiled and accepted that as a good enough reason to resolve a draw, and then she asked me which breeds of horses were especially multitalented and versatile. "Arabians," I started. "Morgans."

"Morgan." She repeated it, savoring the taste of the word. "Do Morgans come in chestnut?"

"Yes."

That settled it, and her new Ranger was christened Morgan. That truck would serve well and faithfully for years, outlasting Mom herself at Erdenheim. He was a manual, which I have trouble driving because of an old knee injury that makes me a little slower than I'd like on pedal switching, but since I was about to head off to college, we both agreed that it didn't make sense any longer to include me in her car equation. I already had plans beyond college, my life mapped out, and Mom herself fully supported those plans and believed they would indeed be my path.

How things can change.

That first long trip in Morgan, taking me from southwest Missouri to Minnesota to college, was epic, and Mom and I often laughed about it later. We even laughed about it that night eventually, once events progressed past frustrating to absurd. We were late getting started, but neither of us wanted to miss the target time at college the next day. She figured that even if I couldn't split the driving, I could provide company to keep her awake, and so it was that we set out in late afternoon, planning to drive through the night instead of the original version of doing most of it that day and then stopping at a motel and finishing up in the morning.

The first leg of the journey went smoothly, and we stopped for a meal and break at my dad and stepmother's house in Kansas City. Rena, my stepmother, offered to go with us as another driver to spell Mom both there and back, but we really wanted the trip to ourselves, and she understood.

Half an hour out of Kansas City, the heavens opened, and a deluge began. The windshield wipers were struggling to keep up even on high. Still, we splashed on, figuring that we would drive out of it. We did, but that took us six hours—six hours of the heaviest rain I've ever seen.

A little ways on through the storm, Mom suddenly came to attention and looked in the rearview mirror, then at the sides. "Something's wrong with this tarp," she said. "It's torn loose or something. It's flapping more than it was." All of my college-bound possessions were in Morgan's bed, and we had bought a brand-new tarp to go on top, as well as brand-new rope to criss-cross clear over several times and tighten the tarp down to the truck, tying the rope to large S-hooks attached to the bottom of the frame.

Mom pulled over, and we got out to check. It was like standing underneath a waterfall; we were both drenched before we even reached the bed. We could find no specific fastening that had pulled loose, but the whole thing definitely wasn't as tight anymore. We had just checked the load at Dad's before leaving Kansas City. Odd that it had pulled loose all over that quickly, but that was the only explanation we could see then. With stereo shrugs from our respective sides of the truck, we tightened the rope all around. Meanwhile, of course, freeway traffic whizzing by was courteous enough to splash us. Satisfied that the tarp was tight again, we returned to the cab of the truck.

We were just starting to progress from drenched to merely very damp when Mom looked in the mirror and slowed. "It's loose again." I checked my watch; we had made thirty minutes. We pulled over again, got out, and stood once more in the pouring darkness as we retightened that rope. Passing traffic still showered even more water on us. We pulled the rope as tightly as we possibly could, giving it our full weight, then got back in. I rode turned around and watched it suspiciously out the back window for the first few miles, but it was tight.

At first. Around forty-five minutes later, the tarp was once again visibly breathing and tugging at its moorings, slowly gaining altitude. We again got out, still in the storm, and again tightened things up. We then stood there looking at it accusingly for a moment in spite of the rain, just daring that rope to loosen again before our eyes. It seemed to be behaving itself innocently, and we got in and drove on, making it another thirty minutes before we once more had to stop.

The answer struck both of us simultaneously. "This rope is stretching." In the dry first leg of the trip, it had held firm, but once the heavy rain started, it kept stretching. Clearly, that fiber stretched when wet. Neither of us had thought of checking how the rope held up in water when we bought it. Mom and I looked at each other across the truck bed in the pouring rain, two drowned rats constantly being splashed by the passing traffic on the interstate. (The whole night, not one driver stopped to offer help.) Then both of us cracked up. Standing there holding on to the truck bed, impossibly wet yet still somehow getting wetter, we laughed until we cried. "Smile, Deb," she called across Morgan. "We're on Candid Camera."

At this point, it was late enough, and we were between cities enough anyway that we weren't likely to be able to replace our rope soon. My belongings so far were holding up remarkably well, most of the clothes in trash bags, and the tarp had never completely come undone at any edge thanks to Mom's noticing right away and putting us on guard. Still, we couldn't keep progressing down the road in thirty-minute increments. I'd be lucky to get to college by midterms at that rate. On the other hand, this rope was becoming ever more useless and obviously wasn't going to help us out.

Mom rooted around behind and under Morgan's seat, looking at the few things she had already put in the new truck, but there was no other rope. There was, however, a nearly full roll of duct tape. She hadn't meant to leave that in the truck, had just needed one piece for something a few days earlier, but never had gotten around to taking it out, and it had rolled under the seat.

That duct tape was our salvation that night. Taking the rope completely off and giving up on covering the whole bed, we shrouded the tarp around a central bundle of my collected stuff. Then we used the entire roll of duct tape around that tarp, wrapping it thoroughly in all sorts of directions. We just hoped that the duct tape, applied wet, would hold. We stopped for a prayer as we got back in the cab, and I'm convinced that no two people ever petitioned the Lord more fervently on behalf of duct tape than we did that night.

It held. We got out an hour later to check, just in case my view backwards in the dark wasn't completely reliable, but the bundle was as neatly secured as it had been at first, and the tarp was still tight.

Just as the rain stopped, as the dawn after that long night—a night in which sleepiness definitely was not a problem—started to break, we finally passed a hardware store. We looked at it, briefly toyed with the idea of waiting for it to open, then drove on. We had more faith in duct tape by that point than in any type of rope. In fact, from then on, it would become a staple of every trip, and Mom and I would ask each other before heading off to anywhere, "Do you have duct tape?" Then we'd laugh, reliving it all. It was a lousy trip in a lot of ways, but it remains a treasured memory. Start to finish, we were in it together.

Mom made good time once the rain stopped ("Morgan wants to gallop!"), and we arrived at the college only an hour past noon. I checked in, and it took both of us a good thirty minutes to untape that large tarped bundle in the truck bed. We could feel the looks and unspoken questions of other parents in the parking lot. "Do they have that tarp fastened with *duct tape*?" On my own, I might have explained, but Mom always took pride in appearing odd when the oddness had a good reason behind it and wasn't just for its own sake. Once we got down to the prize in the center, we found all of my things relatively dry and in remarkably good shape considering. Together, we hauled them up to my dorm room.

Then it was time to say goodbye. Mom had pre-pared her parting words, I'm sure, and probably had rehearsed them a few times, but she didn't give me a typical Polonius-style flood of advice. There was no advice at all. Instead, she simply said, "May your wings be strong," then turned and walked away.

I loved college. The work was hard enough to chal-lenge me, and I threw myself into it full speed. The school wasn't known as a party school; while there were a few on the wilder side, study was in fact the goal of most students. My idea of a good party had always been curling up with a book, so I fit right in.

Mom and I spoke on the phone at least once a week, long conversations that were remarkably bilateral. They didn't strike me as especially bilateral then, just as us, but my roommate once commented on it. "She talks to you as much as you talk to her. She actually asks your advice herself on things instead of only giving you advice you didn't ask for. My mom isn't like that."

We also discussed my classes, and she enjoyed fol-lowing them at a distance. I majored in English. The two vocations I had tossed around for consideration as a child had been teaching and being a veterinarian, but teaching won out. I had always felt drawn to teach, and I loved words and good literature.

However, I also disliked kids. I fully believe that my maternal instinct was either left completely out or switched to animals. My dolls in early childhood were never my babies; they were characters in stories. Wanting to avoid prolonged exposure to kids, I knew I could never teach in the public-school system. I would have gone crazy in one day flat. There are people with the gift of dealing with children, and I admire them tremendously for it, but I'm simply not one of those people.

All of this combined to create a well-thought-out goal: I would go on from this excellent but undergraduate college to another to get my doctorate. I would then teach English at a university, one which also focused more on learning than parties and one carrying enough of a price tag that students there had a serious stake in this and would be more likely to apply themselves.

That was the plan. Along with that plan came a timeline. I've always liked timelines and definite goals. At the age of eight, I charted out the entire week broken into one-hour blocks, made up a schedule including everything, responsibilities as well as free time, and posted it on my closet door. Then I truly followed it. Mom was amused. She wasn't waiting for me to break it or thinking it was a fleeting phase; she just enjoyed the fact that I had decided to do that myself.

That bent for planning, for charting things in black and white and then working life out accordingly, was something that I would have to learn to release on and trust God for, especially later as we progressed into Mom's illness.

The original timeline as I saw it in those college days involved me being well established with tenure in a teaching position and also being able to buy my farm by age forty. The farm was a dream Mom shared: my farm, always my farm, but she would eventually wind up living there herself and be the landscaper. Each of us would occupy her own house but side by side. Her planned presence at the farm had nothing at all to do with possible failing health or decreased acuity; we just wanted to live together eventually and share the mutual enjoyment of the land and each other.

It was in college that the farm of the future, as yet unspecified, acquired in advance the name of Erdenheim. The word means "earthly home," and I ran into it in German class one day. One of my favorite verses has always been 2 Corinthians 5:1: "For we know that if our earthly house of this tabernacle were dissolved, we have a building of God, a house not made with hands, eternal in the heavens."[7] Erdenheim. Earthly home. The residence for this earthly moment, though not for eternity. So I named the farm Erdenheim, and Mom and I would talk about it often, considering what we wanted to plant or build there, wondering what the details of the land would be. Of course, we couldn't peg things down too much until we actually knew the land and its features, but it was fun to dream together.

I had a job at the library, part time when school was in session, full time when not, and that, too, I loved. There also were a few vacation weeks off from that job, though never the entire summer. In between junior and senior year, Mom and I took a driving vacation together during those weeks while Daniel stayed with Grandmother and Granddaddy.

We went first over to North Carolina, then up the East Coast, stopping in to see Michael in Norfolk, on up to New Jersey, then turning across Pennsylvania, and finally finding our way back home. We took Morgan—and duct tape!—but encountered no problems. Ten days in a Ranger or in a tent at the campgrounds at night, just the two of us in perpetual tight quarters, and we still weren't tired of each other's constant company by the end. On the night of my twenty-first birthday, we were in Pennsylvania, and Mom took me out to eat at a restaurant in a large old building that still had cobblestone floors and originally had been an inn. Yes, we were told; George Washington had indeed slept there.

The train of my plan for life chugged along as I had intended right up to the second part of senior year. Then it derailed. At the time, I couldn't explain why and had no idea what God might be up to. He slammed the door on my postgraduate plans so firmly that the echoing thud resounded. No possible misinterpretation; I was not meant to go on to graduate school. At the time, I was not angry but bewildered, wondering what on earth had gone wrong, worrying what I was supposed to do next. I have given thanks for that roadblock many times since.

I was offered a job in Minnesota that I wouldn't have minded, not teaching but working with books. However, while I had loved the education, four years of Minnesota winters had been more than enough. With graduate school off the agenda, I simply moved back home, though I did pay rent from that point on while I lived with Mom.

Stuck with a degree with honors but without the further graduate work that would have been required really to use it professionally as I wanted, I started looking around for a job. In the meantime, Mom, who was medical office manager for an internist, asked me to do the transcription. Their office transcriptionist had injured her shoulder and would be out several weeks. I had no experience at all with transcription, but I was a good and fast typist already. I well remember my high school typing teacher telling us that this would be one of the most valuable courses in our entire education. Mrs. McClure, you were right.

Mom had worked part time often at transcription herself to supplement her full-time medical office positions, and she assured me that I would pick it up quickly and that she could help me. So it was that I started typing for a living. I also purchased my first car, since I couldn't drive Morgan. I found another job at a hospital in medical records after a few months, and life ticked steadily on.

A year after my return, the doctor Mom worked for moved from private practice to employee status at a university clinic, and his office closed. She found a position as office manager with another doctor, but she simply wasn't satisfied. After working with several doctors with whom she had "clicked" professionally, she could never quite get on the same wavelength with this one. He was an excellent doctor; they just didn't mesh. At the same time, the hospital where I was working in medical records and where she had done part-time transcription a few times in the past was having more dictation than they could handle.

It was Mom's idea to go into business together. She had decades in the medical community by then and a good reputation, and she said I had picked things up very quickly those months working in her office. She predicted that with more mileage, I would become quite good at this before long, and she could help on the front end of the learning curve. We decided to start a medical transcription business, working as an independent contractor for the hospital, adding other accounts as we could. Plotting out the figures over a celebratory Chinese dinner at a restaurant one night, we concluded that yes, we actually could make this work.

The business was named Two-by-Twice Transcription. Two-by-twice is an old term meaning occupying a very small amount of space, and that definitely fit our first "office." It basically was a widened hall, barely holding two small desks, with routes to the bedrooms running straight through it and a water heater that always felt like a third person supervising in the corner. Mom quit, I quit, and we went into business on our own.

We did consult initially with an accountant used by several doctors she had worked for over the years. He approved our figures and planning and gave us business tips. We definitely didn't want to incorporate and get into that more complicated field, and he explained that a formal partnership agreement was not technically a requirement to having a partnership. It was nice to have but would cost more to set up, and the main purpose of one, according to him, was protection of the partners against each other in case of a disagreement. Mom, sitting in his office, looked over at me and said, "I can't imagine any disagreement that the two of us couldn't work out by ourselves."

Two-by-Twice was a success, but a growing shadow stretched out across the family as the 1990s progressed. Grandmother's dementia was increasing. Grandmother had always proudly and efficiently managed her life. She was the practical one; Granddaddy, while possessing infinite good intentions and compassion, slipped on concrete details.

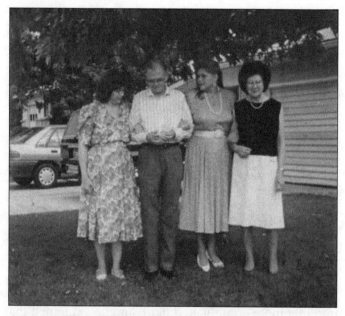

**Mom, Granddaddy, Vicki, and Grandmother at the 50th wedding anniversary celebration.**

When they fell on hard times back in their early marriage, she had gone back to school, earned her master's, and taken a job teaching. The remedial reading program in the public school became her kingdom, and she ruled it efficiently but with unquestionable authority. No student reached her class without already being labeled slow, and in decades of teaching, she never had a failure. Not once. Hundreds of people walk the world who can read because of Grandmother. She never had a failure because she never knew how to give up on anything. If they were there to learn to read, then they *were* going to learn to read. No other outcome was conceivable for her. She would switch from one method to another if needed, but always, ultimately, something worked.

Now that sharp efficiency, that management skill, was running out like water down a drain. She had had to take retirement because her illness was beginning to affect her work. Granddaddy cared for her as diligently as he could, but things finally reached the point where she would have to be placed in a facility.

Mom spent a few weeks going to different area nursing homes, interviewing and inspecting, collecting data. One thing working in the medical field teaches you in a hurry is that not all doctors or facilities are equal. Much better to drive farther to a good nursing home than to pick the one next door simply because it is next door. No matter how often you visit, the staff there will spend more time with your loved one than you will.

In the end, the nursing home that earned Mom's highest approval was only six miles from Grandmother and Granddaddy's house. Grandmother was placed— she had efficiently purchased long-term care insurance years before—and Granddaddy was able to drive up to visit her daily.

Mom and Vicki also visited regularly. They alternated Saturdays, and each week, after the visit, they would talk on the phone and update and support each other. The whole local family came several times a year. We had long celebrated all occasions at Grandmother's house, from Christmas to birthdays, and we moved those parties to the nursing home, meeting there as a group every month or two. After one experience of trying to bring a fully cooked Thanksgiving dinner from multiple locations over an hour away and still keep it hot, we usually settled for sandwiches and chips, but we did our best to keep the family gathering around her just as we had celebrated previously.

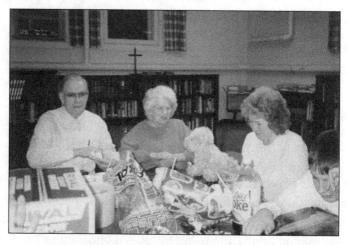

**A family celebration at the nursing home with Granddaddy and Grandmother.**

Watching Grandmother's decline was painful, I'm sure much more so for Mom and Vicki than for me. She had been so efficient, so competent in her life. She just faded away.

It was during this time that I began to realize why I had to come back home. I was needed here. Mom talked to Vicki weekly, but she discussed the situation in detail with me all the time as well. I also kept our business going on days when she was accompanying Grandmother to doctor's appointments or going down to meetings. Mom never missed a doctor's appointment or a care plan meeting. She and Vicki had agreed that based on their respective fortes, Mom would be in charge of the medical oversight and Vicki the financial.

Mom needed me beside her. That was enough, more than enough, to wipe out the disappointment and bewilderment. I still wasn't sure where my life was heading long term, but I knew I was where I was supposed to be at the moment, and being certain of that made it all right.

It was in the context of Grandmother's illness and the subsequent early hints of Granddaddy's that Mom told me one day that I was the best friend she had ever had. "In fact," she continued, "you're such a good friend to me that sometimes, briefly, I can forget you're my daughter."

I count that as the highest compliment she ever gave me. Not everybody has; some, on hearing that line, thought it awful that a parent could forget a child for even a second. But to me, what it said was, "Even if there was no biological relationship, even if you weren't part of my blood family, I would value your contribution in my life. I would choose to know you. My esteem for you isn't only because we're related." It was a compliment.

Life wasn't entirely consumed by Grandmother and by the business, of course. The old interests and personality were still there. Mom remained perpetually surrounded by cats. I had my own cat by this point, my first Siamese, bought just because I'd always wanted one, but Mom continued to favor the scraggly, hungry, down-on-their-luck waifs who appeared at the door and applied for adoption. Wherever she lived, all her life, they did appear at the door. We used to joke that the Statue of Feline Liberty stood in her front yard bearing a slightly modified inscription that read, "Give me your tired, your poor, your huddled masses yearning to eat free."[8]

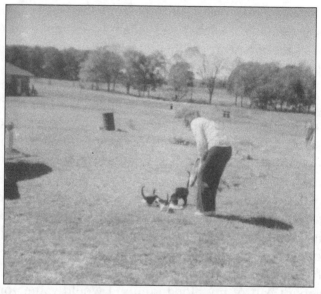

**The patron saint of hungry cats.**

Books were another constant. Mom had a scientific bent and read things like Stephen Hawking and hard physics. For recreation, she loved science fiction and fantasy. She appreciated literature, but when she just wanted a mental break for a while, it was usually science fiction. We also had family movie nights, with Mom, Daniel, and me gathering with popcorn in the living room each Friday evening. She also read the Bible regularly, of course, and we had many wonderful debates on points therein, often disagreeing but always doing so civilly.

Her driven personality carried forward to how she read some verses. For instance, she truly believed that when we were given dominion over the earth, this applied by extension to creations of humans—i.e., things like computers. When a computer was acting up, to Mom, it was challenging her God-given authority over it. To me, obviously things created by people would be less well crafted than things created by God, so problems could be expected to arise. Not to Mom.

Her own body would similarly annoy her. She had an old knee injury from one day years before when she had decided to attempt water skiing at a work picnic by the lake. Typically for Mom, she fast-forwarded over half of the instructions given by the doctor who owned the boat, and she called, "Hit it," before she was set and ready rather than after double checking her position first. She had her skis crossed, and the resulting flip as the boat accelerated injured her knee badly, though we never knew exactly how. No X-rays, no CT scan. She simply took ibuprofen, used home exercises, gritted her teeth, and pushed on, and it slowly over months improved. But it would ache with weather later, as would a hip she had sprained once, and when it was annoying her, she would stand one-legged on the offending extremity for several seconds "to teach it a lesson." She still was slaying lizards.

One year in the 1990s, the three of us went down to Silver Dollar City to the fall arts and crafts festival, something we tried to do every few years at least. That visit, she found an oil painting that she fell in love with. The artist accepted monthly payments, and she purchased it, easily her most expensive day ever at Silver Dollar City. Normally, we just walked around and looked, enjoying that in its own right, but she simply had to have that painting. It is a scene of a dark-haired girl, probably early teens, swinging on a homemade swing made with long ropes and a board seat. The rope is strung from a high, overarching branch of a large tree, and the girl is swinging way out into the air, almost too high, with legs kicked forward and head thrown back. The atmosphere is pure joyful abandon. Mom named it "Flying" and said that the girl reminded her of herself.

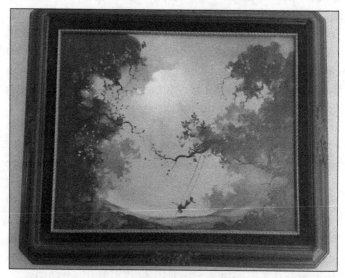

**Flying, original oil painting by Vincent Fleming. Used with permission.**

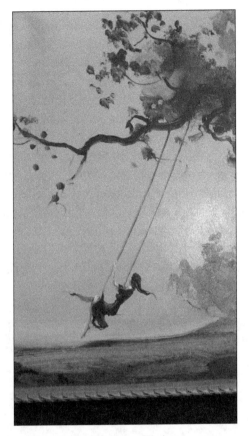

**Detail from Flying.**

Music was another constant, and it was one we could better share now that I was old enough to be in adult choir myself. Mom loved choir. She approached it like that girl on the swing in the painting, giving it every ounce she had. I remember the pure passion she threw into her singing. We usually stood next to each other in the choir loft, and I learned her subtle body language that was too far away to be visible to the congregation. The way she leaned forward minutely into key changes; Mom and I both loved key changes. The way she would gather herself before a difficult spot. The way her little finger would crook slightly a fraction of a second before a high note, as if reaching out to touch it physically as she sprang for it vocally. At times with intense music such as the "Hallelujah Chorus" or the wonderful final rising swell of "The Majesty and Glory of Your Name," she would actually have to remind herself to breathe. She could get so caught up in the piece that she would forget. And on finishing an anthem, she would lean just slightly toward me, not actually turn her head to look, which might have been distracting for the congregation, but give the faintest tilt in my direction. It was an irrepressible exclamation of the soul, thrilled at the privilege of sharing the music together, a silent, "Wasn't that wonderful?"

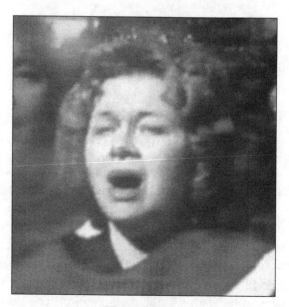

**Mom singing.**

She also loved handbells. I never got much into bells, but Mom was a faithful member of the handbell choir and went to events with them. She occasionally ran into Rena at these, who was attending with the handbell choir from her church in Kansas City, and they would make use of the opportunity to chitchat. Mom and Rena always got along very well, and Mom sometimes would jokingly refer to Rena as her "wife-in-law."

One member of the church told me later how at one such bells event, when that lady became ill, Mom insisted on leaving the festival early and driving her a few hours back home. She had Morgan on the trip that day because the church van couldn't quite hold everybody. She monitored the other woman all the way home and made sure things were stable before leaving her. Always, when faced with a true need, Mom would do whatever she could to help others.

Mom became deeply involved in music for local nursing home ministries. She would sing hymns while another church member played organ or piano, and then a retired missionary in our church would preach. Several times a month, she participated in services in one nursing home or another. She also sang to Grandmother on her visits, of course.

Another outstanding musical memory is the game that Mom and I played during duets. Singing duets with Mom was especially fun for both of us. We had nearly identical singing voices, just two more notes on top for me. We also could sing low as well as high, and sometimes, we would play with the listeners by flip-flopping parts. I would start on soprano with Mom on alto, and at the end of a phrase, we would switch. We kept that up several times in a song, and we would watch people try to figure out which of us was singing which part. Even for other musicians, it was hard to differentiate. At other times, we sang it straight and held each part all the way. I am so glad that I have audio recordings of a few duets and several more recordings of Mom singing solos.

I never made a conscious effort to collect recordings of her; whatever I have is not from luck but providence. I always thought there would be more time; she only turned fifty in 1994. Grandmother had not started failing until well into her sixties. I never dreamed that those 1990s would be Mom's last good decade.

I have replayed things countless times since, wondering what I might have missed in those years. I'm sure I did miss some signs before late 1999, when I first was sure. She was a little sharper, a little quicker, a little shorter at times. But she was also under stress with Grandmother and, by the end of the decade, with Granddaddy added to the mix. At the time, I put anything I noticed down to the stress of dealing with her parents' illnesses. Probably much of it was, but probably not all.

Two more things of import happened in the late 1990s before I saw the writing of Mom's future illness on the wall. First, I was asked by a man at the church to substitute teach his Sunday School class one day when he was going to be out of town. I had never taught Sunday School, had never even considered teaching Sunday School. I think that on some level, I always automatically thought of kids in that context, and teaching kids would have been a disaster. My patience with them was nearly nonexistent, and they, having remarkable radar, would have picked up on that right away.

But teaching a class of adults simply hadn't occurred to me. I protested at his call, saying that I wasn't sure how to teach Sunday School, and he replied that he thought God wanted me to do it. Sometimes, we need a friendly shove from someone else to change our perspective. I agreed to give it my best shot for this once, and I spent a few worried days during the rest of that week preparing.

I absolutely loved it. I not only loved it; I felt fulfilled in it. I felt like a puzzle piece snapping into its predesignated position. The adult class members enjoyed me, too, and I started teaching regularly when I had the opportunity.

It only occurred to me later that perhaps *this* was what I had felt drawn to. All those years, I thought I wanted to teach at a university, a desire that had had the door slammed on it, a desire that, as soon as I realized I was needed at home, had disappeared. At that point I wouldn't have taken such a position even if it had been available to me. But maybe I just had the focus a little off, like an optometrist's lens, and it needed another turn to reveal what I actually was called to do. God knows what he is doing, and in fact, I hadn't lost a calling by changing career paths.

The second landmark of the late 1990s was that I found Erdenheim. Mom and I had been through three rental houses together since my return from college, but the last of those had a pasture attached. I had promptly brought my current horse home from the stable where he boarded, and of course, he needed another horse for company. The herd grew, and when we had to move again, I realized that I couldn't afford to board them all. I needed a place with some land, and Mom needed a house in the same school district for Daniel, and we agreed that lightning wasn't apt to strike twice and again provide both of those in one location.

So I started looking around farther afield, while she focused on the school district. I found the farm one damp and dismal day in March. It looked nothing like I'd imagined, and I recognized the land at once. Even muddy, even with outbuildings having trouble holding themselves up, even with an entire list of faults, it spoke to me. Had it been in good shape, I couldn't have afforded it. I rented it for the first months, then bought it.

I turned thirty in 1999. Mom gave me a birthday cake that said, "Welcome to the better side of 30!" In talking one day shortly after that, she was the one who pointed out that I was ahead of my original goal. On the initial postgraduate plan, I had wanted to be on Erdenheim by age forty. With my own plans collapsed, with me back home being a support for her, God had given me my farm a full decade earlier. I was reminded of the verse, "He will give you the desires of your heart." Rarely on your timetable, sometimes, as with the teaching, not quite the same desires you once thought you had, but he will give them. Sometimes, you even get them sooner.

1999. Even now, saying the year sounds to me like tolling bells or like the solemn opening of Rachmaninoff's splendidly moody *Prelude in C-Sharp Minor* (with, as always in my memory, that still-echoing cry of "FISH FEATHERS!"). For most of it, the last whole year. I wish I had known.

Many years later, after Mom's placement in a care facility, I found a few old videos of the choir and skimmed through them with full painful hindsight. I have no video of Mom singing a solo; I'm fortunate to have as much audio as I do. But there were those few services, many of them cantatas that we had recorded on old VHS tapes. I watched them, looking for Mom, catching glimpses in the pan of the camera, each one a treasure.

It was in the Easter cantata we did in 1999 that the camera paused and held for several seconds on the two of us. We were side by side, singing together. I froze the recording and took a screenshot. The resultant picture quality wasn't great, but the shot was priceless. Mom throwing herself fully into the music, giving it every-thing, flying. Me next to her. Easter 1999, the last one in which she seemed to me to be fully herself.

Just ahead waited not lizards but dragons.

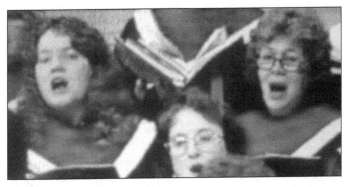

**The two of us singing in the Easter cantata, 1999.**

# 4.

# *"If I Forget..."*

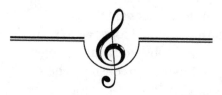

I n late 1999, Two-by-Twice changed transcription
program platforms to stay compatible with the hospital that was our main client.

Some people simply cannot handle technology, even
with their full mind and abilities intact. Granddaddy
was one of these. He never could learn to use an
answering machine, and while Mom once gave him a
subscription for an episode-of-the-month tape series of
*Gunsmoke*, his co-favorite Western along with *Bonanza*,
he couldn't seem to get the hang of the VCR and didn't
watch them unless we were there to run it. She told me
that he had never been very quick on mechanical points.
Granddaddy's forte was people; he was a born pastor
and shepherd to his flock.

Mom, however, was good with new inventions, and
her mind never had a problem grasping a change in procedure. She had her first cell phone before I did, and
she loved it and began using it regularly immediately.
She enjoyed science and new frontiers. Computers
and machines annoyed her at times by challenging her

God-given dominion over them, but she had never had difficulty learning the basic ropes.

When Two-by-Twice started, I still was working out my notice at the hospital when Mom met the tech folks delivering our first TeleStaffer. They spent a few hours that afternoon training her, and she picked it up at once, even though she'd never before used a piece of equipment remotely like that. She subsequently taught it to me a week later. Twice more over the decade, we had added equipment or programming that required a significant change, and it was like shifting gears in Morgan for her, just dropping into the new one and going on a little faster. She enjoyed technology and progress, as long as it cooperated, and when it didn't, she was ever ready to discipline it back into line.

1999 was different. Ominously different.

The software vendor sent one of their field representatives out to provide training and orientation, and we received three days' worth of her along with the purchase of the software. The rep installed it on our work computers and then began teaching us the program.

Mom couldn't get it. Not only that; her frustration suddenly seemed fragile, not determined. All her life, everything about her had been forward, charging full speed at obstacles, slaying lizards. Never before had I seen her simply shrink from a challenge and concede failure without putting up a fierce fight. Now, she stated in near tears that she guessed she'd better go get a cardboard sign and sit on street corners begging for donations because she was *never* going to understand this.

Our field rep, a neat lady we both enjoyed talking to, even suggested staying more days simply for Mom's sake. That would have cost us more, but beyond that, by the third day in, I knew that something was *wrong*. Truly wrong. There wasn't any possibility I saw for such a radical change other than the fact that her own mind was starting to fail. The writing was on the wall. To preserve her privacy, I asked the rep to stick to the planned schedule and said I would keep working with Mom more slowly. She departed with a cheery, "Don't worry. Some people have more trouble with technology than others."

But not Mom. Never before Mom. By the time the rep left, I was certain that Mom herself was in the early stages of dementia. Like both of her parents, she was walking that long, dark road into mental fog, even if still several mile markers behind them.

Once we were alone, I started trying out techniques. Mom was still extremely functional in life. This was going to be difficult, but I didn't think yet, at this early stage, that it would be a complete failure, and she needed for her own pride to still be able to work. I broke it down. I wrote up notes. We tried mastering *one* thing, just one, per day. Today, we will learn how to connect to the hospital. Tomorrow, we will learn how to log into the system (a separate step from connecting and one that failed completely if done in the wrong order; that was a very common error). The next day, we will learn to request a job. Her computer monitor sprouted a veritable forest of Post-it notes. The actual typing itself, well established for her for decades, wasn't any problem once she was in a job. The issue was purely the software the work was framed in, navigating the system, requesting jobs, reaching the hospital data-base to set up demographics and patient information, sending completed reports. Slowly, painfully slowly, it all began to gel, and finally, she was working again at near her old speed.

I didn't mention my new conclusion, not then. Nor did she mention her new fear, though it was painfully present in her eyes as she doggedly and bravely forced herself to learn the new program. Those days had to have been a shock to her even more than to me. Later on, she would be in fierce denial of any mental decline, but at that point, she had too much of her mind intact to avoid the glaring conclusion. I believe that both of us saw the shadow of the future by the end of that year.

She was only fifty-five.

Her parents continued their own walks into the mental sunset, and I was struck then by something that I'd notice more strongly later with Mom: even with the same diagnosis of Alzheimer-type dementia, there were individual differences. Grandmother seemed to fade down to a wisp. Her last year or so was basically in what I thought of as rag-doll phase. She almost never spoke and simply was there, propped up in her wheelchair by her lap buddy or tucked into her bed. They fed her, washed her, and dressed her. In the years prior to reaching that phase, she did have either a couple of hallucinations or just mental returns to yesteryear in which she apparently was teaching school again. These moments were not disturbing to her in the slightest. "She always was in control of her classroom," Mom recalled. Grandmother would point at an invisible student and say, "Now, I see you back there, passing notes. Sit up and pay attention!"

To the end, she had the family strong will. Her death in the early 2000s was dragged out to an incredible degree. From the time the nursing home told us this was it and we were most likely down to hours, she hung on for a full week. Defying all medical data, in total kidney shutdown even though on IV fluids, she lingered. Mom and Vicki rotated shifts that week, trying to keep someone with her, and I ran the business and, a few times, went down to give Mom some company. We would sit and sing, picking old hymns that Grandmother had loved, and watch her, counting breaths. While we were there, another always came. "She never did know how to give up at anything," Mom said fondly.

Granddaddy was a completely different case. In addition to his memory starting to decline, he did have some paranoia crop up fairly early in his presentation. Prior to his placement, he worried about Vicki and Mom handling the finances, even though he had been lousy at finances all his life. Before her illness, Grandmother had managed the household for decades after his own failure at it; that wasn't a prior independence that he lost at the end. His driving also became more of a concern. Mom finally talked him into a complete neuropsychiatric evaluation, and she asked me to come along with her to the results session. "I want a witness in case he challenges this," she told me.

We sat there in the office, the three of us, and Granddaddy heard his sentence. To Mom's relief, he accepted it bravely, though he was obviously rocked. She had feared a scene in the doctor's office; fortunately there was none. He agreed that very day to placement in the nursing home. At first, we rented him one of the apartments on the campus with nurse visits and supervision of medicines, but the nursing home itself quickly recommended moving him to a unit in the full facility. He was a wanderer, and after several rounds of them having to call the police to find him when he had walked off and gotten lost, it was clear that he needed a higher level of care.

From that point on to his death many years later, he lived in the nursing home and wore a WanderGuard. A worker at the nursing home would tell me later that her strongest memory of him was him looking around furtively as he went through the doors of the building when leaving with Mom for a doctor's appointment or, in the early days, for just a lunch out. She said he always wore an expression of half guilt, half pleasure at making his getaway and would pick up the pace just a little as he went through the doors.

He was in his disease course more mobile much longer than Grandmother and also more talkative. He still wandered on the different wings, even though he couldn't leave the building without triggering an alarm. He was one of the first patients moved to their locked dementia unit when construction on that finished. As he ambled pleasantly but determinedly through the unit, he would pick up all sorts of things and say, "I've been looking for that." Then he would hide them in places, such as in his sock drawer underneath the socks, lest someone steal this treasure. Mom and Vicki, visiting on alternating Saturdays, always cleaned out his drawers and returned his loot to the staff for redistribution to its rightful owners.

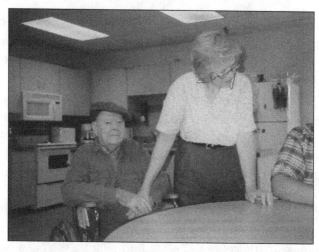

**Granddaddy and Mom at the nursing home.**

Grandmother and Granddaddy were not roommates because he was prone to innocent but unknowingly dangerous things, such as trying once to cut her eyelashes with nail clippers. His helpful impulses and devotion remained, but his judgment was shot. Once the locked unit was built, though he moved there, she did not. He was an amiable wandering kleptomaniac who needed the stronger security; she was a rag doll and no management problem by then for anybody.

When Grandmother finally did give in to death, it was on one of Vicki's watches. Mom did no work for that entire week after and wasn't up to her usual production for quite a while when she restarted. She kept apologizing for dumping the business on me alone, and I kept telling her it was perfectly okay and understandable that she needed some time to grieve. Grandmother's loss hit her extremely hard.

It was about that point that I asked her what she wanted at her own funeral. She wanted her body donated to a medical school; Mom was always interested in science and was nothing if not pragmatic. "I'll be done with my body," she said. "If anyone else can get some good and some education from cutting it up, they're welcome to it."

She did leave specific instructions for the music at her eventual service. She wanted her two favorite hymns, "Great Is Thy Faithfulness" and "We're Marching to Zion," but she was determined that "We're Marching to Zion" should be done *right*. While she loved the hymn, she never requested it during favorite hymn nights at church, as she disliked how congregations sang it. I can hear her voice now. "It's a *march*. It's upbeat, positive, *forward*." She could give a great rendition of the typical church version. "We're crawling to Zion, mournfully dragging to Zion, we're creeping upward to Zion, the beautiful city of God."[9] At her funeral, she demanded, we were to sing it as it should be sung, and I promised to carry out her wish.

I couldn't quite promise her one other request, but I said I would do my best. She had loved the song "No More Night" since the first time she heard it. It became her favorite solo about heaven, and she relished the beautiful words, especially in relation to her parents' illness. The text recalls the great promises of Revelation 21:4: "And God shall wipe away all tears from their eyes; and there shall be no more death, neither sorrow, nor crying, neither shall there be any more pain; for the former things are passed away."[10] She asked me to sing that song at her funeral. I wasn't sure that I'd be able to make it through that right there in her service, and she said she'd understand if I couldn't.

I watched her closely during those early years of the decade, viewing everything now with newly opened eyes, and the mile markers of that dark road became a little clearer as they loomed up into view. She slowly became less tolerant of things, such as a doctor's incorrect grammar in dictation or typos in a newspaper or a bulletin. She used to just be annoyed by these, shrug the errors off with a pointed remark, and move on; now, they approached another campaign to slay lizards at times. She said more than once that she was going to march down to the church office and offer to proofread the bulletins or volunteer at the newspaper for the same. She never actually did, and really, we didn't have an unusual amount of typos. Everyone has one now and then.

One Christmas, in the cantata, there was a song carrying not only the words but the title of "Jesus, You Are Him." The composers needed it to rhyme with Bethlehem. I thought Mom was going to blow a gasket. Not only did the choir receive over a dozen lectures on proper grammar during rehearsals, but every time Mom sang that line, she corrected it to, "Jesus, you are *HE*!" Yes, even in performance. Not only that; she accented it, firing it as a defiant arrow aimed at the composers who dared to break grammar for the sake of rhyme scheme. She also fumed about that song through all songs before and after, either anticipating or remembering it. Mom in her prime would have brought it up once in choir practice but then consigned the error to the list of annoying things that you couldn't change because you couldn't control others. It certainly wouldn't have ruined the whole cantata for her. Not this time; this error became another lizard that demanded slaying with full ceremony. For her to use music of all things to make an aggressive assault on such a minor point rather than losing herself in the pleasure of singing as usual was very odd.

I don't remember the exact year, but I think it was around the early 2000s that another and much more pleasant musical memory of Mom was formed. The choir had a Christmas banquet, and one of the party games of the night consisted of the pianist picking a carol from the hymnal and playing only the first note. The floor was opened for guesses, after which she would play the first two notes, then the first three, and so on until someone named that tune. Mom was unbeatable. They finally disqualified her to give others a chance. While she was in the game, I only remember once that she required three notes. Most of the time, she could name the song on two and name it quickly, not even pausing for consideration. Twice, remarkably, she nailed it with only one note. The woman who had been that little girl reading and rereading the hymnal during church was in her element playing that game.

Her memory was failing, but the signs were subtle, though increasing slowly. I'm sure that they weren't even noticed at this stage by most people. I doubt I would have noticed as early as 1999 myself if we hadn't been partners in the business and working together all day. Driving especially worried me, and I kept a very close eye on her driving, making it a point to follow her from work to church on Wednesdays or at any other opportunity. As far as I could tell, though, she was still at this point a safe driver, and she wasn't getting lost yet.

Only once in those years did something about her handling of Morgan jump out at me, and when it did, it wasn't subtle. Even a child would have thought something was wrong that night. It was a day in early spring 2002, and I was out at Erdenheim. I had something to leave for in just fifteen minutes, but I was ready, and hating to waste fifteen minutes, I decided to test a few fence posts. I was gradually replacing fence, but a lot remained to do. In testing fence posts, I would grab a wooden post and try to shift it, attempting to judge if any rot had made its hold in the ground less secure and whether it would require replacement. I did have safety glasses that I wore when removing old wire or applying new, but I didn't pick them up that night. I wasn't going to be working with the wire; I would just test a few fence posts as a wedge to fill a slight schedule chink before something else.

I never made it to that evening's planned event. A couple of fence posts into my efforts, I reached a post where, on the firm shake, an old, rusty strand of barbed wire snapped. It speared me in the right eye. I have a high threshold for seeking medical attention, though Mom's was higher, but that accident crossed it from the first moment. Blood was running down my face, and there was no question in my mind that I needed prompt emergency care.

Going back to the house, I called Mom. I still remember her cheerful greeting before she knew something was wrong: "I was just thinking about you." I told her I had hurt myself and needed a ride to the ER, didn't think I needed to be driving with my eye like that. She told me to stay put, and she would be there in the soonest possible jiffy.

It was more than a jiffy from the city to Erdenheim, but she made excellent time. As we drove back, almost to the interstate, she suddenly noticed Morgan's gas gauge. It was sitting on E. She had meant to fill up the next morning, thinking she wouldn't need to go anywhere else that day. The trip clear out to Erdenheim hadn't been in her figures. The gas was low enough that we decided she'd better stop for gas on the way to the ER instead of after, since running out of gas on the interstate would hardly have helped my situation.

So she pulled into a gas station, got out, and looked at the pump in absolute bewilderment. I was still half seeing red and hurting besides, so it took me a moment to realize something was off here. "What's wrong?" I called.

She shook her head and stamped one foot in frustration, a quirk that Grandmother also had shown under extreme pressure. "This thing won't *work*," she protested.

I got out and went around to study the gas pump with my good eye. She hadn't even taken the handle off the hook yet or pushed any buttons. "You have to pick where to pay first," I said.

Mom seemed totally baffled. "Where to pay?" Though computerized pumps were fairly new, this was far from the first one she had seen; she did these exact same steps weekly at her favorite station and had never had a fight with one.

Concern growing, I indicated the screen. "See where it says pay here or pay inside? You pick which one you want."

"Okay." She hit pay here, then waited, looking at the total cost. The figures hadn't started moving yet, of course. "It's still not working."

This was scaring me, and I could tell it was scaring her. She was trying hard to keep calm, but she couldn't make heads or tails of that screen. I broke it down, as I had with the computer program in 1999, and she required each step. "You put your card in. Right there in the slot. Okay, now you pick which octane you want. You like to give Morgan midrange. Then you pick up the pump handle. Now you open the fuel door. Take off the gas cap. Okay, put the nozzle in. Now squeeze." She followed the instructions for Gassing Up Your Car 101 obediently, but at no step did she anticipate the next one. The computerized pump had completely scrambled her, leaving her mentally adrift.

Once Morgan was full, I told her to replace the nozzle and the fuel cap. When we were back in the truck, I watched carefully, but she started up at once, shifted gears smoothly as she pulled out, and headed for the interstate, stopping correctly at a light as we approached. The whole rest of the trip to the ER, she didn't put a foot wrong driving, but all that way, I was recalling that day many years prior when my foot was badly infected and she took me from the stable to the hospital in Leonardo. She had been smooth, pure efficiency in very similar circumstances when one of her children required help in a medical emergency. This night was the second example I had of that scenario, and she clearly wasn't her former self. Years later, there would be a third comparison event, and her decline would be immeasurably worse by then.

Mile markers on the road to dementia. I grew to hate them, but I couldn't help watching them go by, reading each one, and yet I could do nothing to stop them.

That same year, 2002, my first book was published. I had published a few short stories and poems before, but this project was definitely the largest undertaking to date. The church turned 150 years old in 2002, and I had been commissioned the year before to research and write a sesquicentennial history. The book took me a year to research, a few months to write from notes after that, and I loved every minute of it. History has always lit my fire in the same way that science lit Mom's. I was forced for the first part of those 150 years to rely solely on archives and research; for the second part, in addition to records, I interviewed the longest-term members of the church who still had their faculties intact. It was fascinating, hearing all the old stories, weaving them into the fabric of words. Mom attended several of the interviews with me, but she didn't participate, just enjoyed listening from the sidelines.

Mom was my proofreader and critic. I have been glad for that many times since. She saw my first book and was helpful in the process. Not too many years later, she still would have been able to read it but wouldn't have been a good editor, and several years after that, she wouldn't have been able to read it at all or to understand it if she could. But at this point, she was still able to give me her critique.

Mom had always been a wonderful person to bounce writing off, and I often had sent her stories or poems I had written in college. We shared a love of words, and she also was entirely honest. That was what I appreciated about having Mom read something

I had written: she truly gave me her evaluation of the work. There wasn't a trace in her comments of, "I love this just because you're my daughter and you wrote it," and I didn't want there to be. That kind of feedback might be good for refrigerator art for a child, but for someone who wants to become a serious writer, it's not the response you're looking for. Mom not only could tell me what she liked—and, more rarely, didn't; she could explain why and was enough of a writer herself to have good radar. Some of her suggestions I took, some I didn't, but the genuine and knowledgeable opinion was always appreciated. She loved the church history and read it chapter by chapter as it moved from my head and notes into the pages.

It was also in 2002, in the fall, that I joined the Mid-America Singers. This group would become an incredible support for me on the road ahead. A semi-professional auditioned community chorus, they sang music of a difficulty that took everything I had, that caught me up in it, letting me lose myself and forget the struggle at times during those rehearsals. Paradoxically, it simultaneously could sharpen up the situation and bring it into more poignant focus. Music is such an incredible language, taking pieces and emotions that are tumbling over each other and recasting them into order, sense, and ultimately resolution. I truly think that without the music I got at church and through Singers, I would have gone insane myself in the coming years.

Sometimes, a piece done by either church choir or by the Singers would seem written directly to me. One of these from church was "An Expression of Gratitude," which starts out quoting Philippians 1:3: "I thank my

God in all my remembrance of you."[11] Yes. I would say that verse sometimes to myself and later to her even on the lowest visits. I would use it in the tribute video I made for her funeral, and always, I would hear the music, establishing and expanding on the words. So many other songs through the years reached out to me, reminding me that music still is present and often at its best in difficult times. In the darkest valley, there is music for that. In the longest night, there still is music for that.

But greatest of all, if I had to rank them, as a musical expression of my own journey during her illness was a song the Singers did in late 2004. The words came from the works of Robert Browning, well-known English poet. His wife, Elizabeth Barrett Browning, was also a poet; she was the one who wrote the sonnet that begins, "How do I love thee? Let me count the ways."[12] She was mostly an invalid from age fifteen on, and her health was a constant third member of their marriage. Robert Browning knew what it was to be a constant caretaker. He knew what it was to give your best and see a loved one fail anyway. His wife's problems were physical; her mind remained clear. Still, he lived the decline over years as he faithfully ministered to her. He was there at her death; her last word was "beautiful."

I've always loved the writing of Robert Browning, but I had never run into these particular lines until the Singers performed a musical setting of them in a concert. These words were written earlier than the long ordeal with his wife's illness, but still, the unshakeable faith his character voices here touched me. I was blown away from the first night we opened the score at rehearsal. I felt that those lines might have been written just for me.

I have never sung anything, anywhere, that for me so completely nailed a caretaker's journey, anchored in faith, through a loved one's extended illness.

*If I forget, yet God remembers.*

*If these hands of mine cease from their clinging,*

*Yet the hands divine hold me so firmly,*

*I cannot fall.*

*And if sometimes I am too tired to call for Him to help me,*

*Then He reads the prayer unspoken in my heart*

*And lifts my care.*

*I dare not fear, since certainly I know*

*That I am in God's keeping.*

*Shielded so from all that else would harm*

*And in the hour of stern temptation,*

*Strengthened by His power.*

*I tread no path in life to Him unknown.*

*I lift no burden, bear no pain alone.*

*My soul a calm sure hiding place
has found.*

*The everlasting arms my life surround.*

*God, thou art love. I build my faith on that.*

*I know thee, who has kept my path*

*And made light for me in the darkness,*

*Tempering sorrow so that it reached me
like a solemn joy.*

*It were too strange that I should doubt
thy love.*[13]

Hundreds of times, it must have been, those words
and that song would come back to me over the years.
I would find myself repeating my favorite lines under
stress. The one about being too tired was a prime candidate, but most often when I didn't have time to mentally
cover the whole song, it was either the first line — "If I
forget, yet God remembers" — or that incredible image
almost at the end: "Tempering sorrow so that it reached
me like a solemn joy."

Sorrow tempered into a solemn joy. Yes. Such an
awful disease, but such good memories from before
it, a relationship I wouldn't have traded for anything,
even knowing the future. Even during the later illness,
there were now and then what I thought of as diamonds,

bright moments glistening amidst the black coal of those days, catching and radiating points of light. The years were horrible, exhausting, painful, tragic, indescribable at times, but they were not hopeless. Even at the worst, just when it was needed most, there would come a diamond in the present or a precious memory from the past or a golden thought of the future, and I would be carried on a little longer by a greater strength than my own.

Mom's decline continued, and other people were starting to notice or at least suspect. Her memory failed slowly. Her driving so far was holding up except for that one night when she forgot in the crisis how to gas up the truck. She had no problems driving down to the nursing home on her Saturdays to see Granddaddy. She did start getting lost a time or two in the city, even on well-known routes. This was infrequent but concerning.

She also started showing a little paranoia. The first example of this happened on a visit to the dentist. She'd always had bad teeth but had an excellent relationship with her dentist until his retirement. When she went to another, she finally on his recommendation had all her troublesome upper teeth pulled and had an upper denture and a partial lower created. I remember the day she returned from that appointment commenting how smooth and even her teeth felt and how well they fit. At first, she liked those dentures.

Over the next few years, the story gradually changed. At first, she protested that they did not fit so well and never had, then that the office didn't know how to adjust them, then that they had been made incorrectly in the first place by an incompetent dentist or his unskilled apprentice. Then the story transformed to them being deliberately made incorrectly by a sadistic dentist who specifically wished to cause her pain, gradually adding the reasons he had for selecting her in particular to exercise his grudge upon. The story kept expanding and even finally involved sinister (and nonexistent) special X-ray techniques used as instruments of torture. It almost sounded like one of her science fiction books by the end. Ultimately, she carried her dentures around in a coffee cup, only inserted them for meals and public, and would go into a tirade at the mere mention of the word *dentist*.

Her work efficiency was also dropping. Her accuracy hadn't yet been affected, but her production gradually braked over a few years until, from a starting point of doing about half each of the work with Two-by-Twice, it ran more like an 80/20 split in my favor. She couldn't help noticing that, as we kept daily logs from which to run the bills. When we had to change computer systems again in 2003, the learning period for the software was even harder and more prolonged than in 1999. The growing difference between her line counts and mine was glaringly obvious. She would apologize and present excuses—a lot going on, had a cat crisis come up, something with Daniel, errands needing running. She never admitted the real reason, and we still until the last year of business split profits evenly.

There was one time, only one, when we had an open conversation about her illness prior to her move to Erdenheim. It was in early 2004. I was typing one day on the work and thinking, and as she walked by my desk, she stopped abruptly and inquired, "What's bothering you lately?"

I considered, weighed the day so far—a good one for her—and took the plunge. "You are developing memory problems yourself."

She stood there looking at me for a moment, and then she nodded. "I know." Two short words with a jagged Everest of meaning between them.

I was surprised but relieved, having expected to be challenged. "It's not too advanced yet," I continued, "but it is slowly getting worse."

"I can still do things right now," she agreed. That wasn't defiance but her best effort at an objective assessment.

"Yes. I want you to know, when...when it does get worse to the point where you can't, I'll..."

She put a hand on my shoulder, an unusual gesture. I have never particularly been a toucher, and Mom always respected that. "I know you'll do your best, Deb. I haven't got any doubt of that." She gave me a brief squeeze, then turned away. "Now, where did I put that piece of paper?" She went on about her task of the moment, and I sat there breathing a silent prayer of gratitude. One short, priceless conversation. As it turned out, that was the only one ever conducted between us that calmly and in full agreement, but still, there was that one. A good memory from progressively worried days. A solemn joy. A diamond.

In the summer of 2005, Michael got married, and the three of us went to the wedding. Fortunately, this was held not on the East Coast where they lived but in Melanie's home town in Illinois, roughly a five-hour drive for Mom and Daniel, a little less for me from Erdenheim. We agreed to take Daniel's car, the newest and most passenger friendly, and I met them bright and early at a commuter parking lot on the interstate about twenty miles along, a shorter drive for me than going clear back to Mom's house that held Two-by-Twice in the city. Daniel had worked late the night before due to an inventory at the bookstore where he was employed, and he hadn't gotten home until the wee small hours. He was visibly tired but running on Starbucks. On the way up, we switched off drivers a few times.

The wedding was beautiful, although there was an unforgettable moment beforehand when the glorious, five-tier wedding cake collapsed. Emergency repairs were made by Rena and a few other ladies, and the eventual version, while shorter and a bit rough at the patched icing, was presentable enough.

After the wedding, during the photographs, we got one of my favorite posed shots of Mom. All four of her children were there, something that almost never happened. We gathered on the steps in the front of the church, Mom standing on a lower level wearing her corsage, we children fanning out two on each side behind her. The shadow of her illness was beginning to reach her face, but for the most part, she still looked like herself.

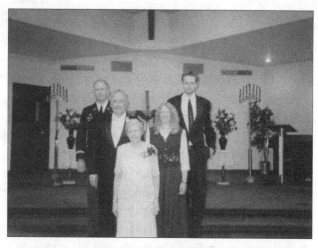

**Mom with all four of her children at Michael's
wedding in 2005.**

It was late afternoon when the reception concluded,
and the three of us paused before starting off to consider
drivers for the return journey. Daniel quickly removed
himself from consideration, saying he was too tired and
sleepy. That left me and Mom. With a very full day
already, darkness approaching, and with St. Louis in
the way between us and home, I wasn't sure she was
quite up to this one anymore, but it would be a long
drive just for me, and she couldn't help but realize that.
She spoke up while I was still diplomatically framing
the suggestion. "I really don't think I'd better drive on
the way back. With it getting dark and all the traffic,
I..." She paused, her eyes admitting the sober fact that
her words couldn't. "Would you mind being the sole
driver going home?"

"No. I think that's a good idea." I climbed into the
driver's seat, Daniel into the passenger's seat, which
was required for his long legs, and Mom in back. We

started off, and Daniel indeed slept much of the way. Mom wasn't too far behind him. That was another change I had noticed. When she wasn't driving herself, she could fall asleep much more easily in a car than she used to.

I drove home, watching the interstate approach and pass one headlight length at a time. Darkness and just a little bit of light. I didn't like this current road we were on in life, but I knew I had no way of changing it. I started singing mentally, not actually aloud for fear of waking my two passengers. My first selection that night out of the current thoughts was the old hymn "Lead, Kindly Light." I've always loved the words to that one, though Mom had said they were a bit too challenging for her personality for her to fully appreciate. "Guide thou my feet. I do not ask to see the distant scene. One step enough for me."[14]

Without realizing it at first, I switched mental soundtracks at some point, and the next time I emerged from thoughts to notice the words, it was Robert Browning. He kept me company for the final miles driving home through the dark.

"If I forget, yet God remembers."

# 5.

# *Moving to Erdenheim*

Erdenheim sits atop a north-south ridge. I get spectacular, unblocked sunrises and sunsets both. As 2005 wore on and shadows lengthened in Mom's life, mental sunset approaching, I began to think more about the farm and our plan that she eventually would come to live there with me. Daniel was out of school now, so the requirement to stay in a specific school district no longer applied.

I was getting more worried about her functionality in the city. Her driving, as best I could judge, was still safe, but she started getting lost more often. She still was leading the music in nursing home services twice a month, and one day that summer, she left Sunday School early as usual to drive over to the nursing home where they were having the service. It was a drive she had taken a hundred times. She had been doing that particular nursing home service since the 1990s.

This time, the familiar road turned into a winding maze, and she got so lost that she completely missed the service and drove around the city for forty-five minutes instead. She finally did find the nursing home just as the concerned organist and preacher had finished the service and were helping residents back to their rooms. Back at her house, she reported this misadventure promptly, phrasing it as "Morgan got lost." She also assured me several times, as if subconsciously reassuring herself, "I wasn't scared. Just kept driving. I knew we'd get there sooner or later." The organist, a good friend who had dealt with her father's dementia, suggested quietly that they ride together from now on "to save gas." Mom agreed.

Two-by-Twice was also a concern. I was carrying the vast majority of the work now, nearly ninety percent, and there was no way to deny this. Furthermore, Mom's accuracy started slipping badly. She had a quality audit in late summer from our main client, who was no longer the original hospital we had started with but a large national transcription company contracting for several hospitals. These quality audits were a routine requirement every quarter; you had to maintain ninety-eight percent accuracy. Mom always had previously, even after the symptoms began in 1999. Her efficiency and speed had tumbled, but her accuracy had remained untouched until now. However, on this audit, she scored eighty-two, far, far below minimum. She was immediately put on two-week probation and had to send all reports to Q (quality review), and Q sent her feedback on each one.

She never made it through her two weeks. The feedback she received annoyed her no end; she would fume and read their comments out loud to me. I saw some of the reports myself, and while Mom was missing major medical terms for the first time, those oddly were not what concerned her. No, she was irritated at the objections to her hyperediting of the doctors' grammar. I tried to tell her that she was going far beyond her place as a transcriptionist, that she was not just correcting major mistakes but editing style. It was a medical report, not a work of literature. She snapped back at me that it was her duty to educate the doctors. As for the major medical terms she confused, by far the larger concern, she simply ignored those. "Everybody misses a word now and then."

Her feedback from Q became more pointed, and she correspondingly became more defensive. Her halfway audit after the first week of probation dropped into the seventieth percentile, heading the wrong direction.

It was then that Mom decided that "they're trying to push out all independent contractors and only have employees." Yes, it was all a conspiracy by the company. She doubted that she was even making the mistakes in terminology they showed her; they must be inserting those and sabotaging her reports. The fact that I wasn't having similar problems with quality audits fell by the wayside. One day, she squared her shoulders, pointed her chin defiantly, and declared that she would just quit, that she wasn't going to let them draw out the process of disposing of her.

I agreed, realizing that major hospital multispecialty transcription was no longer possible for her. For the sake of the patients, she needed to stop. Typing more slowly had carried no risks except to our bottom line, but her current errors could impact medical care. They also would have horrified her (at herself, not the company) just a few years previously.

Firmly fixed in her "resign with dignity" fit, she composed an email giving notice to the client, and then she nearly wound up in tears fuming that it wouldn't send. When I got from my computer to hers to see what was wrong, I realized that she was typing "Management" as an email address. I don't mean formatted as "management@wherever," which wasn't even the correct address of her supervisor anyway. She was using the sole word Management in the recipient line of the email headers, and of course, the program shot an error message back at her every time protesting that that was not a valid address.

I gently tried to explain that she would have to use "supervisor's name@theclient" as an address as it appeared on the supervisor's emails to her, and she objected that that wasn't correct business letter format. Just because the doctors and the client and the rest of the world used words incorrectly, she didn't have to join them. She got so wound up about it that I had to let her fail a few more times until she gave up (something Mom in full health never would have done). At that point, I changed the address myself on her screen and sent her resignation letter on. The company promptly replied stating that two-week notice wasn't going to be required and that she simply could stop now since she had decided to quit. I didn't blame them.

That left me, however, with a dilemma. Two-by-Twice still had one small client besides the big one, and that account was simple office notes for the doctor she had been medical office manager for until he had closed private practice in the early 1990s. That account she could probably do for a while yet, as it was much less demanding work, and his style and dictation habits were so familiar to her, but the income from that client was very small. Meanwhile, I still was typing for the big client. They hadn't dropped us; they had dropped her. The business income as a whole wouldn't fall much beyond its dementia-adjusted level of recent years, since I'd been doing most of the typing lately anyway.

Still, I already had decided months ago that when Mom had to stop typing, or practically stop typing, I was going to have to back off myself and let the business die. I hadn't expected it quite this soon; Mom's accuracy did not slowly decline as I had anticipated it would. The quality audits were too regular to have missed it. No, she had made a sudden nosedive downward. That moved up the timetable a little, but it did not change my conclusion. Two-by-Twice had belonged to *us*. It had been Mom's concept to begin with; she was very proud of being a business owner. For her own dignity, I couldn't continue our business solo too long with her left on the sidelines merely watching. Nor was any other job still feasible for her. She had reached the end of her working life, and I knew that the little account, the far-simpler clinic dictation, wouldn't last much longer.

Christmas was approaching in a few months, and I chose it as a marker. I would quit myself and try a few other gigs. I didn't tell her, but I always had in the back of my mind that I could return to typing in the future if other areas didn't work out. I knew that our big client would welcome me back at any time, and I could become an employee, working just as myself, not as Two-by-Twice. After a good-length break, it wouldn't be as hard on Mom for me to go back to typing, not as obviously a solo continuation of our old partnership. I hoped I wouldn't have to. I was ready for some variety myself after years of this, but whether I had to return to typing later or not, the business we had built together and run for well over a decade was to be another casualty of her illness.

So I gave her a double-sided statement of Christmas plans. First, I intended to quit typing myself. She enthusiastically agreed, stating that since the big client was on a campaign to kick out all independent contractors, it was only a matter of time until they started a vendetta against me, too. She did insist from that point on, after she quit and during my last months of typing the big account, that we no longer split profits fifty-fifty.

The second part of my proposal was that I would give her a mobile home for Christmas and set it up at Erdenheim. It would have to be a used one, nothing like Chesed. That was the name she had given in advance to her eventual house, the one that she wanted to build on the farm someday. Chesed is a Hebrew word usually translated as mercy or loving-kindness. It is used in the end of Psalm 23: "Surely goodness and mercy shall follow me all the days of my life."[15] Nothing similar to that dwelling was financially feasible right now, but a used trailer would be a suitable home for her, albeit a simple one.

Mom was thrilled and grateful. Through the remaining few months until Christmas, James and I both gave her some money each month, enough to pay rent and the power bill. She accepted. So it was that Mom mostly retired. She began to spend more and more time reading politics and current events on the computer. She'd always had the interest, but it would become near an obsession in her final computer-literate years. I still drove into the city every day myself to type at her place and to keep close tabs on her.

She did not, by the way, file for Social Security. She was only sixty-one at this point, but she didn't even file once she could have. All her life, Mom held very firm opinions. Once she got an idea fixed in her head, even preillness, it took dynamite to shift it. She had long been convinced that Social Security was a Ponzi scheme and that if run in that manner by anyone except the government, the managers would have been prosecuted years ago. I thought she had somewhat of a point, but she carried it to the max, as Mom usually did. Having concluded that the program was not being morally run, she refused to participate by drawing from it. Whether or not you agreed with Mom's convictions, you couldn't deny that she did have the courage to live by them.

We started looking at used trailers advertised for sale. Some we saw were unbelievable. One had multiple holes in the side, not little holes but holes that you easily could have used as supplemental doors for people. Another was missing the official doors; several were missing windows. Mom and I stood in yard after yard of flotsam and jetsam and eyed mobiles with extremely open-air ventilation and tattered insulation hanging out around the edges, and we just looked at each other. Dementia moved to the back seat; our silent communication in those moments was as crystal clear as it ever had been.

After several false starts, we found it. The trailer was older, obviously not with limitless life left, but it had been well maintained. I thought it had the years needed still in it. The owner was a pleasant and interesting woman we thoroughly enjoyed meeting, a disillusioned landlady who, after the escape while owing rent of her latest tenant, was ready to quit the whole game. The price was reasonable. Erdenheim had been paid off earlier in 2005, well under a decade after I had bought it, but I was remortgaging it for some money to use in setup of the trailer and life reshuffling. Moving that trailer, rewiring it, and the electric contractor work wound up costing much more than the trailer itself, but I believe it was the one we were meant to purchase for Mom.

The only real concern Mom had was that the trailer had a gas furnace. She was still rather jumpy on the subject of fire, always remembering the house fire in Georgia, but she was even more uneasy with gas. When things go wrong with electricity, your house catches on fire. When things go wrong with gas, your house explodes. The chances of escape are much better with fire. She asked if I could get the trailer converted to all electric, and I said I was sure it was possible. (It was. Not cheap, but yes, possible.) I promised her that for her peace of mind.

On the positive side, the trailer also had a deck, a massive beast built with very heavy wood. Mom loved that deck. I asked the seller if the deck came with the trailer, and after some discussion, we agreed to a contract that stated I was buying everything above the ground. If I could move it, it was mine.

Events clicked smoothly into place like puzzle pieces. I kept busy moving fence at Erdenheim, enlarging the yard to make room for the trailer in the back. A mobile home moving company was booked for the trailer; they suggested December 29. Close enough. I wasn't going to pay extra to have it moved on the actual holiday, even if they would have done it.

Meanwhile, Mom was happily planning and truly excited. I gave thanks again several times that autumn that this move had been part of our long-term plan all along. She didn't have to fight it. It wasn't perceived as a loss of independence or being placed under supervision, even if I in fact wasn't sure she would have been safe much longer in her former home.

With the trailer signed for but not yet delivered, I called a master electrician and explained the situation. He came out to Erdenheim to consider the pole location and the stretch of wire to be run to the site for the new trailer, and he agreed that it was perfectly possible to convert a house over from gas. "New circuit box, new furnace, new water heater, some new wiring..." The mental figures behind his eyes were almost visibly spinning like the price on a gas pump. Still, he had excellent references and qualifications, and his several-thousand-dollar estimate was no more than I had expected.

In the end, as we were standing outside talking, he nodded toward the perfectly flat stretch of land in the upper pasture between the two baby sugar maple trees that I had bought with part of the payment for the history book. "Now *that*," he said, "is a wonderful natural building pad." I agreed but told him the site was taken. I didn't want Mom's trailer there; I intended to build there myself when I was able. The sugar maples would frame the structure a measured distance from each front corner. Many people had been unable to see this farm whole, as it would be; it was definitely a work in progress. But as I pointed out to the electrician this ultimate building site and described eventual plans, I saw genuine enthusiasm and understanding awaken in his eyes. He had the imagination required! He actually saw it!

He definitely saw it. "You'll need electric run out there someday, too," he said.

Box by box, load by load, we moved Mom's stuff into my house. This was driving me crazy, and she sympathized, but at least it was temporary. My house (which wasn't my ultimate house I intended to build, just the old, beaten-up structure that was there when I bought the place) wasn't overly large to begin with. Moving her stuff in on top of mine left it looking like a warehouse with narrow aisles. Still, we had given notice on her rental house in Springfield as of the end of the year. We had to get a head start on moving, couldn't wait until the last two days of the year to transport everything, though the biggest pieces were reserved for a U-Haul then.

A week before December 29, the trailer mover's wife called me to make sure all systems were still go. She said she had to apply for a permit from the state. "We used to be able to do it just a day in advance, but then Jeff City upgraded their computer system, and now it takes about four days to get the permit back." The permit was duly applied for, and now the only remaining question was the weather. You are not permitted to transport a mobile home on the public roads in anything except good weather. December wasn't the greatest season for this, but the long-range forecast at that point looked promising.

The twenty-ninth dawned a bit foggy but with that feeling that it was going to burn off. I drove down to the trailer park an hour away to meet the movers. Mom wasn't with me; she and Daniel were very interested but had suggested themselves that logistically, they probably could help most by staying out of the middle of today's big event. The tow truck and escort vehicles arrived, and we ran into the first complication. When I was asked how many concrete blocks I had at the destination site, my answer wasn't enough for the head mover. Leaving careful directions, I raced off to the lumberyard, and they continued hitching and packaging the trailer.

The second complication came when the mobile lumbered ponderously up the road and stopped at my driveway. My driveway is long but narrow. I had figured they would have to go off the gravel turning in, but I hadn't figured on the tree at the corner interfering. I thought we could just brush through the few overhanging limbs, which weren't thick ones right there, just danglers. With the trailer parked on the country road, everybody surveyed the tree in question, and the man in charge shook his head. Some trees brush through, he said, and some didn't. Naturally, I had the wrong sort of tree. It would damage the trailer, might even rip the roof. Did I have a chain saw? No. Did the neighbors? I started trying to call the nearest neighbors. Nobody who was at home could help; those who might have been able to help weren't at home.

Meanwhile, one of the workers found a Sawzall in his tool box. To me, it looked like the sort of thing that Grandmother had used to carve the Thanksgiving turkey; he said it was useful in odd moments on setups. It wasn't ideal, but it was all we had short of the hand saw. The ringleader stayed on the ground and supervised, and the others took turns climbing and trimming that tree. As advertised, the tree proved amazingly resilient even on little branches. It took well over an hour to cut a trailer portal, and the poor little Sawzall was smoking by the end. For this side show, they added $50 to their fee, and I'm amazed they didn't add more.

Once the way was cleared, the leader took a final look at the eventual site. With the trailer coming in and proceeding around my house in the only direction possible, it would be pointed wrong, but I had thought of that one. A hole was precut in the pasture fence and a few posts removed. I figured he could drive the trailer on into the pasture where he had a world of room, straighten and get his angle, then back it slightly cater-cornered out through the gap again and into place. He nodded, jumped back into the cab, and started off, and I don't think he missed the designated spot by more than two inches. I watched admiringly, used to backing up horse trailers, which can turn stubborn themselves on occasion. I couldn't imagine backing that seventy-foot monstrosity, but he did so smoothly, one long motion, no false starts and adjustments. He fully deserved his status as a professional.

Mom showed incredible patience that day, but she couldn't resist calling just as the crew was finishing leveling and blocking the trailer. "Is it there? Is it done? Can we come out?" I told her to come on, and they arrived an hour later. The trailer was inspected proudly. It had no power, no water, no phone, and no amenities at this point, but it was sitting in the right location. Mom looked around Erdenheim with a happy sigh and proclaimed, "The nice thing about this place is that I'll never run out of something to do." Amen. She soon would choose picking up rocks as her assigned task. I'd been picking up rocks intermittently for years out here already, but there certainly remained enough for her to pick up more without fear of running out.

December 30 was a day I'd rather forget. I had a one-day stomach bug and wasn't feeling well at all, and I also was driving the U-Haul. I hate diesels; the noise of them gives me a headache. The furniture was solidly and stubbornly uncooperative. Mom's piano was even worse than before; we had moved it a few times previously, but between the dementia and my virus interfering, it gained several hundred pounds that day, I think. Once at Erdenheim, I backed up the U-Haul to the trailer door in many jerky start-stops, nothing like the mover's smooth performance the day before with his much-larger load.

Then, after I had turned in the U-Haul back in the city and headed off to the farm that night, Coleridge, my F-150, broke down on the interstate. God works in mysterious ways. Due to me feeling so lousy, Mom had talked me into driving the truck back unloaded that night, the first time in weeks I had done so, leaving the final boxes for another day. Thus, we had no cargo to shift on the side of the road in the dark. She was right behind me in Morgan, and we simply transferred me, left a note on the dash of the truck, and called it a day.

Out at Erdenheim, because it was winter and because the electricity wasn't hooked up yet, Mom couldn't actually move into her trailer. Thus, she temporarily slept in my place on the hide-a-bed portion of her couch. Just the hide-a-bed portion; it had been unbolted from the couch itself to lighten things for moving. For future reference, she didn't recommend sleeping on naked and unsupported hide-a-beds. She was at least a step up in accommodations from Daniel, who had to make do with a sleeping bag back in my office. The first night, after he rolled it out and then went off to do something else, one of my cats moved in during his absence and erupted in a feline fury as he climbed in later to go to sleep.

The electrician arrived. God got the lights turned on in one day; the electrician took a few weeks. The project was punctuated by emergencies elsewhere, but he really was quite diligent. There was simply a lot to be done. Meanwhile, after a few days, once Coleridge and I were both well again, Mom and I returned to the trailer park to pick up the deck.

The deck was waiting for us on its side. The trailer movers had disconnected it and flipped it back to allow the trailer to move away, and it lay there with the steps reaching skyward, looking like the corpse of some pre-historic beast in full rigor. My original plan had been to unbolt it into a few easily haulable pieces, but we quickly modified that. Flipping it back right side up only confirmed the weight of it, and unbolting the steps took a few hours on its own. It would take too long to disassemble the deck floor even partially. With the steps off and then the railing removed, I considered the remaining deck, large and flat and perched on six legs. I measured it mentally against the full-sized bed of Coleridge.

"I doubt it," Mom replied, hearing the thought. "It's too big."

"Not by much," I countered. "We couldn't get both sides of legs in; it's too wide. But if we put one side of legs in the bed and let the other legs hang over the outside, I don't think it would shift any." We had come armed with a rope—and with duct tape, of course, just in case.

Mom considered, then nodded slowly. "If we can get it up there. Tally ho!"

"Tally ho!" I agreed, and into the battle we plunged.

I treasure the memory of that day. The two of us fought against that deck, working together, coordinating effort with unspoken understanding, on the same wavelength as we so often had shared. It was brutally hard work, but we went at it with strategy, not just force, and inch by inch, we won.

Halfway through, with the front of the deck in/on the truck and the back still on the ground, we took a break and walked down the road to a convenience store for a Coke and a snack. We had no fear of the deck toppling during our absence; the whole afternoon, it had shown no inclination at all to move, not even with help, certainly not on its own.

The walk was about half a mile each way, which Mom did easily, keeping right up with me, wanting to go faster if anything. I would remember that journey to compare her walking to just two years later. There and back, we talked about Erdenheim, not about her increasing issues but about the future, immediate and long term. I knew already that a good bit of our speculation would never come to pass, but still, I soaked up the moment. I wasn't sure how many days were left in which we would be so completely in sync, working perfectly in double harness as had been routine for us in her prime. That day, we still had it, fully partners.

With the deck finally resting atop Coleridge, one set of legs in the bed and one dangling over, we tried to shift it and test stability. It wasn't going anywhere.

Unloading it would be fun, but I had no fears for our safety on the road. The thing was simply too solid and heavy to blow or move. "That," Mom announced with satisfaction, "was a dragon." I heartily agreed. No mere lizard there.

After driving home, we simply parked Coleridge that night and went on to bed, and the next day, we did it all in reverse. Mom often sang during the unloading, calling on her assorted "project" songs. That day, I didn't join in, just listened.

With the deck finally in place, she wanted more and more to move into her own house, but the electrician was still working on all the wiring. Meanwhile, we began shifting her belongings over. I also did some investigating; we had found Ruth, one of the barn cats, in her trailer a few times even when the door had been firmly closed, so there had to be a hole somewhere. I found the single (I hoped) hole underneath the trailer on the same day that the electrician finished. With the hole patched and the power and heat (electric heat as requested) on, Mom and Daniel moved over for the first night in her new abode.

In the middle of the night, she awoke to the unmistakable sounds of an angry cat. Her own Yeller was on her bed, agitated and frantically scanning the room, but the feline fuming was coming from below. Finally, she realized that it was Ruth, shut out of her designated hole. The cat was cursing directly below Mom's bedroom, voicing her complaint loud and clear to the human audience above. Mom burst out laughing and calmed Yeller, and finally, when Ruth gave up and moved on in disgust, Mom went back to sleep.

It was January 15, a new phase, the start of a very different year.

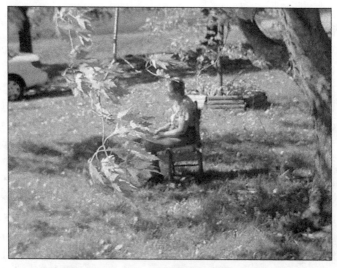

**Mom in the front yard at Erdenheim.**

# 6.

## *Twilight*

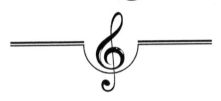

Mom settled into life at Erdenheim with enthusiasm. She raved about the farm, the ridge, the sunrises and sunsets, the star gazing, and, above all, the peace of the deep country. "I want to die here," she often said, and I hoped that she could. She began working on picking up rocks as she had promised, and she started landscaping plans.

Meanwhile, as she prepared for spring, her functionality piece by piece continued its march through late autumn.

Her driving was my major concern, as I tried to determine when that would have to stop. I took every opportunity I could for an assessment, either riding with her or following her, but at that point, I still never saw her do anything unsafe. I did suggest that she no longer drive at night, citing the multitude of deer that inhabited the woods along these back-country roads. That much was true; not a week went by without deer sightings. Mom accepted that limitation and agreed it was a good idea.

In the spring of 2006, Granddaddy died. Mom had told me on Easter weekend that she thought he was knocking on heaven's door, and while there was an extra visit that week, she made no attempt to keep a vigil as she and Vicki had done with Grandmother. I wondered at the time if part of her realized that she herself was no longer up to it. She always had been very close to Granddaddy, closer than she was to Grandmother, but his death somehow didn't shake her up as much. He died late one night toward the end of that week, and the nursing home called to inform us. She hadn't been there, but she truly didn't seem to mind. In fact, she seemed relieved.

That weekend, just a day or two after his death, the Singers had a concert. Mom always came to our concerts, usually coming along early with me, and she would sit out in the auditorium and listen to warm-up and final rehearsal, getting a double dose of the day's program. She was as rapt as that three-year-old spell bound by Beethoven's *Third Symphony* decades earlier.

That particular Sunday, our highlight piece was John Rutter's "Feel the Spirit," consisting of arrangements of seven different spirituals. "Deep River" had always been a favorite of Granddaddy's, but it was the seventh spiritual in the set, "When the Saints Go Marching In," that touched Mom most that day. I watched her as we rehearsed, and I could tell from her face, her eyes, and her smile that she was picturing the welcome party in heaven at that moment. For her, that concert and those spirituals were the prelude to his funeral a few days later.

After Granddaddy's death, the need for those long drives every other weekend to the nursing home, alternating with Vicki, was gone, and I was relieved. She'd never gotten lost on that road, but still, it was quite a distance.

Work was the first area of life to fail completely during her farm years. As I'd feared, the final account for Two-by-Twice, routine office notes by the doctor she had worked for for so many years, did not last long. This was much easier and less demanding than the multispecialty hospital accounts had been, although I had started reading over her work to watch for any decline in quality. I never told her that and just sought private chances.

The breaking point with that last account, however, wasn't accuracy at all, at least not accuracy of the reports she had typed. The client began complaining that a few times, not all reports on a tape had been transcribed, the final one or two left off. The clinic suggested providing a list attached to each tape of the patients whose notes were contained thereon. That way Mom could check off each name as she transcribed the report to make sure all notes were completed.

Mom reacted strongly, as if her integrity had been challenged. The very idea of them wanting her to check off patients on a list offended her. She had done transcription for years and years, and now they had decided that they just didn't trust her. Of course, there had to be ulterior motives. She came up with a complicated scheme of what their actual intentions must be, and I suggested quitting that account, too. Everything else already was gone from Two-by-Twice; that little clinic was the last pulse blip of our business. She agreed; she didn't want to continue doing work for them if they were getting paranoid. Thus Two-by-Twice, our partnership, officially died. Mom had done the first report ever for the business, and she typed the last.

This left Mom totally without income, at least from working. I wasn't charging her any rent on her trailer, of course, but there was still the question of food and utilities. Social Security remained out of the question in Mom's eyes; she could get wound up at the mere mention of the idea. Therefore, from that year through her nursing home placement, James sent her some money each month for living expenses, and she was grateful for it.

That spring I landed a job as a home-health aide, a field that had always attracted me. Working with seniors, listening to their stories, helping them out in their own homes—I absolutely loved it. Unfortunately, the job didn't pay much. At the end of 2006, I did wind up going back to the typing, as there just wasn't enough income, and intangible rewards don't pay the bills. To my relief, Mom accepted that as a step just for me, separate from any identity with Two-by-Twice. I did apply to our former large client, and they were glad to welcome me back as an employee.

It was in the late summer of 2006 that Mom stopped driving. That evening is seared into my memory. Due to especially complex schedules that Wednesday, we didn't ride together to church as usual and simply met up there at choir with the two trucks. This meant Mom would have to drive back late, but the summer evenings were long, the daylight wouldn't be totally gone, and I would be tracking her in Coleridge all the way.

When Mom set off from church that evening, it was like the fateful quality audit almost exactly a year before. Suddenly, precipitously, there was a marked decrease in function. There was also near absence of directional sense; she was totally lost in the city within just a block or two from church. This wasn't a temporary wrong turn corrected later but wild scrambling. Afraid she was heading for Texas instead of Erdenheim, I wound up taking Coleridge around her and getting right in front. She latched on as if with an invisible tow rope, and she followed me on home from that point.

From that advance guard position, I also could manage situations, never putting us in a tight spot, stopping for all yellow lights, making slow turns when one was required, and no doubt driving others on the road nuts. Their opinions didn't matter to me that evening; I was just trying to keep Mom out of trouble and get her home safe and sound. Even so, she tried once turning into the wrong lane at a frighteningly major intersection. Just as Morgan started that way, not drifting but directed, I pulled Coleridge over again in front and hit the horn sharply to get her attention, then moved the angle back and completed the turn into the correct lane. She understood and tucked in on my rear bumper again.

By the time we reached home, I was ready to take the keys from her that very night, physically if required. That was it. She simply was not safe on the roads.

Thankfully, an argument wasn't necessary. She had come to the same conclusion herself, though she couldn't openly admit it. As I approached her after we both parked, she spoke up before I had a chance to open my mouth. "Morgan *scared* me," she worried. "He wasn't acting right at all. I think he's having electrical problems. Or engine problems. Or something." She studied the truck as I studied her. "He is getting to be an old truck," she continued.

Well, if that was the bandwagon she offered, I was perfectly willing to climb on board. I didn't care what she called it, just about the end result. "Yes, he is getting to be an old truck," I agreed. "You know, maybe it's time Morgan retired."

She reached out fondly to pat a fender. "I think maybe it is. Such a good little Morgan horse. But he's getting old."

"I don't think you'd better drive him again."

She nodded. "I don't think I want to. Something's wrong with him."

From that day forward, she never drove again, never even attempted it. We kept a very close eye out for any reconsideration, but regardless of how her mind cast the problem, she never wavered on the decision. So it was that Morgan entered retirement, sitting parked in her side yard throughout her remaining years on the farm.

Another oddity began to increase in the Erdenheim years. Her children, in particular Daniel currently and myself in the old stories, seemed to be becoming younger to her. Time ran backwards. As she recalled events of yesteryear, especially the house fire, I slowly retreated in the story from a young child to a toddler to eventually a babe in arms. She even told me one evening, "Of course, you don't remember, but our house really did burn down once." When I replied that I absolutely did remember the fire, she gave me an odd look. She never seemed to forget that I was an adult now, but in most of her memories, no matter how old I had been at that time, I reverted to infancy.

Her attitude shift regarding Daniel was similar. Daniel had always liked to retreat to his room and close the door when he got home, preferring to read, play games, or watch TV privately. This had never struck either Mom or me as odd, since both of us liked alone time at regular intervals as well. However, she started now to develop a belief that any time he was in his room with the door shut, he was asleep. Even speaking conversationally to her in her trailer would elicit a firm, "Shhh! Don't wake up Daniel!" By her last summer on the farm, it would be impossible to speak above a whisper in her house without being scolded for it. Over the years, I realized that she was reacting exactly as if he were a baby, and she was afraid the world would wake him.

The final time she sang in our church was another mile marker on this road to dementia with no exits before the ultimate one. That last song came on a Wednesday night in 2007. Our congregation had three opportunities during the week for a solo: Sunday morning, Sunday evening, and Wednesday night prayer meeting. Over the years, Mom had been up to the demands of all three, even the televised Sunday morning service. Her music had started to become a little more of an effort of concentration lately, but she still threw her full heart into it. That night, she was to sing at prayer meeting, and a good friend of hers was accompanying her on the organ. They met beforehand to rehearse, and I went on into the chapel early with her just because we always were together at church unless we had separate responsibilities at the moment. We simply enjoyed each other's company. I wasn't checking up on her, not that night. I just was looking forward to hearing her sing.

With only the three of us in the deserted chapel, well before the congregation arrived, Mom began her practice. From the beginning, she was floundering.

This again was an abrupt, sharp decline, not just a slow spiral. I was around her singing in church all the time; it had never before been anywhere close to this difficult. She kept getting lost, even with the music, even on this familiar favorite. She stopped repeatedly and so obviously was getting rattled that I asked if she would like to try doing it as a duet. She seized that idea like a lifeline.

So I joined her on the platform, and we sang together both then in practice and a little later in the service. Gone was our former playful part-swapping. We both sang the melody. I traced the music with my right hand on the page throughout, and she followed it as closely as a map to an unfamiliar destination.

Later, I privately told the music minister that she had dementia and probably was past her solo days. He thanked me for the information and never asked her to sing after that, and Mom herself never brought the subject up again. She couldn't have helped noticing her absence from the lists, but she seemed more quietly grateful than shut out. She continued to sing in choir, but that, too, was getting harder.

It was during the summer of 2007 that I injured my hands, and that night was a painful realization for both of us, even beyond the physical pain of the accident. It was the third occasion, the first two being the blood poisoning in my foot in childhood and the barbed wire eye injury, when I was hurt or sick and Mom had to react regarding transportation.

I was trying to get a business going breeding horses on the side, and the morning of that fateful day, I left the farm early to deliver my two broodmares to the vet for ultrasounds. Due to the aide work that I was still doing part time, the day's schedule wouldn't allow me to arrive at the vet for an appointment when they usually did ultrasounds. Therefore, we had arranged in advance that I would deliver the mares prior to the vet clinic opening, put them in the back corral behind the clinic, then go on to my early aide shift. That afternoon, when I had finished a later aide shift, I would collect the mares from the back corral again, probably after the clinic had closed.

"The best-laid plans...gang aft a-gley," as the poet Robert Burns noted.[16] Which means, as Mom always said after quoting that line, that Murphy's law was active in former centuries as well as this one. On this day in 2007, the first obstacle to my best-laid plans was a deer. Driving through a foggy early morning, I was heading down our country road when a deer popped out and hit me. I didn't hit him; he hit me. He bounced off the front fender of the solid-steel horse trailer with a sharp bang, picked himself up, and raced off in startled retreat. I stopped to check, but other than a small dent on the fender, everything seemed fine, and Kate, the horse under whose nose the deer had attempted to implant himself, wasn't hurt at all, just spooked. I still think that this too-close encounter with the deer was the first link in the chain of that evening's accident.

Later that day, I returned to the vet clinic to collect the mares. They were out in the back corral waiting for me as planned, and I opened up the trailer, deposited a treat in each manger, then collected Kate. This left Freedom in the corral alone very briefly while I loaded Kate first. Freedom always was somewhat of a ditz. She reminded me of the wife on *Green Acres*. She had beautiful foals, but she was silly. Even if I'd tried to load her first, she likely still would have objected to being somewhere solo for that minute or two.

Kate loaded up very well that night, and I had just put the lead rope through the tie ring at the front of the trailer and was about to tie a quick-release knot when there came a loud, metallic bang. Freedom, cantering around the corral in worried solitude, had slipped on one lap and knocked into the gate.

Kate spooked. There is a whole range of spooks on the equine scale, and this was right at the top, the genuinely panicked mental shutdown. This was completely unlike Kate; she wasn't easy to ride, being a tester, but she wasn't at all spooky. I think she must have had a flashback to the deer hitting the fender right under her nose that very morning. She totally lost it and ran backwards off the trailer, and in that split second, I tightened up my grip on the rope instead of letting go.

Bad decision. Very bad decision. If a 1200-pound animal truly decides to leave Dodge, a 170-pound person isn't going to be able to stop her. Eight feet of rope whipped through my hands at high speed, and the sizzle and the smoke actually registered before the pain. Once the pain hit, it did so with a vengeance. To this day, nothing else in my life has ever hurt like that, not even the barbed wire accident with my eye.

I gathered myself, then left the trailer to catch my horse. We weren't far from the interstate. Even though I knew I was hurt, the horse remained the first item needing attention in this situation both for her own and the general public's safety. Thankfully, she hadn't gone far and was over at the gate conversing with Freedom, still a little jumpy but having decided that no horse-eating monster had her on the menu after all.

After spotting her, I took a moment then for a glance at my hands; the burns covered eight fingers with only the thumbs spared, and the right index in particular, having been the top finger in my grip on the rope, was stripped between the middle knuckle and the junction with the hand.

Gritting my teeth and catching Kate, I reloaded her, returned for Freedom, loaded her, and then drove the truck and trailer twenty miles back to the farm, where I unloaded the mares. I did not, that evening, unhitch the trailer. Instead, after feeding the animals (you *always* have to feed the animals, no matter what else), I went inside my place to attempt some first aid to my hands.

A few hours brought no improvement at all. No home remedy even touched it. Reluctantly yielding to necessity, I went over to Mom's trailer. I had already reported the accident when I got home, but now, I wanted to borrow Daniel's car, which would save me having to unhitch Coleridge before I went to the ER.

Mom stood there in her living room, looking at my hands, and the whole thought train was clear on her face, though unspoken. She wanted to help, to do something, anything. She considered offering to drive me herself, and then she concluded that she wasn't up to it and that the best contribution she could make to the crisis was to step aside. I read her expression, and that final conclusion, even though I agreed with it, hurt as much as my hands. In the heat of that moment, she was honest with herself. She knew that she had nothing to offer and would, in fact, complicate the situation. All she said was, "Be careful driving."

Daniel did offer to drive me, but I turned him down because I didn't want Mom left there alone that night with only her thoughts of worry and uselessness for company. Had I really felt unable to drive safely, I would have accepted his offer, but this was now a few hours out from the injury, hours that had included loading the mares, driving the truck and trailer many miles already (and his car would be easier), and doing the evening chores after I got home. I was hurting badly, but as bad as it was, it wasn't getting worse, just steady fire, and I had ample objective evidence that I was functional even so. No, I thought she needed company that night more than I did.

Three trips for me to the ER, three different mile markers, widely spaced measurements of Mom's decline. Worried efficiency for the first but smooth speed, meeting the crisis straight on, dealing with it: Mom in her prime. That night years later when she forgot how to fill up the truck, confusion briefly overpowering efficiency. This final night, when she knew and admitted to herself that her efficiency no longer existed. These were the thoughts running through my mind along with the pain as I drove to the ER that night.

I saw that realization repeated for her many times over the following weeks. My hands were bandaged for quite a while; it was months until that last and deepest spot, the right index finger, completely closed and the bandage was removed. That right hand has never been quite the same since, which is my own fault. The deer may have started that chain of dominoes, but I ended it. I should have let go of the rope. During those months of convalescence, every time we would get in Coleridge together to head for church or the store, every time I drove us someplace while holding the steering wheel gingerly in my burned hands, I saw the thought again in Mom's eyes. She could no longer help me or make this situation easier. Better for me to be driving injured these days than for her to be driving instead. Not once in all of it did she offer to drive. Her conclusion was unspoken, but her face said it all.

There was another element of car trips with Mom that steadily increased. She continued to fall asleep more and more easily in a vehicle. Formerly, we would chitchat while driving or simply be quiet together, both alert and aware. Now, she was usually asleep before halfway to church. Later on, she would be out within five minutes of starting. Road trips were overwhelmingly soporific.

The Rachmaninoff concert with the *Second Piano Concerto* occurred in September 2007. Mom loved it and was lifted for those moments out of the disease. No confusion, no faltering, no falling asleep there. That night was a priceless diamond glittering from the darkness of her increasing illness.

As the autumn advanced, her walking drastically started slowing down. This was quite a sharp decline measured against events. In late September, we walked down a few flights of stairs from the parking garage and then almost a block along the street to the concert hall. Her rhythm was off slightly, but she made the journey without problems.

Just over two months later, in early December, our progress across a parking lot, no stairs involved, was painfully slow. Mom herself said she just was developing arthritis, but the speed of onset still seemed remarkable. Later, her walking would improve significantly and decline significantly in turn over the years, ebbing and flowing like a tide, no rhyme or reason to it, and well before the end, I decided that it must somehow be influenced by her mental state. It was as if her body was presenting problems because her mind couldn't admit where the true illness lay.

Over those last months of 2007, she did gradually stop going to church choir and then became irregular in church attendance itself. She still was able to sing in the choir, and while it was more of an effort than in her heyday, she never had a moment of floundering lostness as she did on that last attempted solo. But she often simply didn't want to go. I wondered if she didn't want others who knew her well to see her. The decline was unmistakable now with close friends.

In the beginning of December, the Singers gave their annual Christmas concert. Mom went eagerly to hear the Singers, riding in early with me, and that was the night I mentally timed her across the parking lot to the building and compared her speed to that just two months earlier. It was easily ten times slower. She might have had difficulty getting there, but once we were in the auditorium, she settled down as usual and soaked up the music as we practiced. Mom always was so focused listening to music, every inch of her absorbing the notes. That had never changed; from age three to that night in December 2007, she was spellbound by the glories of sound.

By then she could get lost in buildings going to the bathroom, and I was careful to settle her in a seat where, when I was on the risers, she would be in my line of sight right over the director's shoulder. That way, I could keep an eye on her while we rehearsed and go searching if she left for an unreasonable amount of time. The Singers concerts were in a smaller facility and drew a smaller crowd than the symphony, and Mom still seemed to enjoy them and didn't get too nervous with all the people.

After the final preparations came the concert itself. The second half of that particular concert consisted of several of the more popular choruses from Handel's *Messiah*, a work Mom had always adored. (The only bumper sticker I can ever remember her having was on Leonardo: Classical Musician, Handel with Care.) Bringing up the end position, of course, the finale for the whole evening, came the "Hallelujah Chorus."

Not needing the music score for that one, I watched Mom instead throughout the piece at the same time I was watching the director. As with the Rachmaninoff, the great work swept the dementia away temporarily. Her face was glowing, her eyes alight, her expression pure bliss. Like the girl on the swing, she was at that moment flying.

Neither of us knew that night that it was the last, that she never would attend another musical performance of any kind other than what groups visited the nursing home. Therefore, the "Hallelujah Chorus" that evening was the last piece she ever heard at a concert.

I have often thought that had she known, had she been permitted to choose, the selection would have remained the same.

# 7.

# *Powerless*

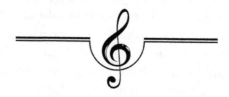

February 22, 2008. A date that personally will live in infamy.

I was over at my place doing transcription that afternoon when my email chime sounded. I shifted programs to see a new message from Mom titled Power Bill. "You don't have to pay my power bill after all. I already paid it."

I was puzzled at first. The power bills for both of us would have been paid routinely in the next week, and Mom knew that. It was her single largest bill each month, especially in the winter. However, I had trouble seeing how she could have paid it. She had no debit card and no transportation, and I was managing all her money. While I gave her an accounting, she never had much money in her own hands. Therefore, I replied to the email asking her how she had paid it.

Her response came promptly. She had paid in cash. I knew she only had a few dollars in cash, certainly not enough to pay a February power bill.

The slow extraction of details through several emails revealed the following story: Mom had been outside working on picking up rocks (an activity she hadn't done in about a year) while I was at an aide shift. A relative from Arkansas, home state for Grandmother and Granddaddy as well as Mom, pulled up in a car in the driveway. Mom recognized him immediately, though she hadn't seen him in decades and hadn't been close then, and they began chitchatting. He was just passing through, only dropping in for a few minutes and had somewhere else to go that evening. She mentioned that the power bill needed paying (during this five-minute conversation with this relative she hadn't seen in years) and that she was worried about getting there to pay it, since she couldn't drive.

The relative promptly forgot that he was in a hurry and offered to take her. So she collected her cash (no explanation was ever provided for the cash), got in his car, and he drove her to the power company's new main office building (which was about thirty miles away and to which Mom had never been). She went in and paid cash to the woman sitting at the receptionist's desk. The woman told her that she didn't need a receipt. Mom just accepted this (which would never happen) and went back out. The Arkansas relative then drove her home, thanked her for the visit, and left.

There were so many obvious holes in this story that I had no doubt that it had never happened. I gently asked if she was sure. Maybe she had dreamt it? She responded as if insulted. She couldn't believe I was calling her a liar. After all these years, I simply didn't trust her. No, it really happened, and the power bill was paid, so I didn't need to pay it. Period. Furthermore, if I still tried to pay it in spite of her having done so already, that would be incorrect management of her money on my part. She expected it not to appear on her financial accounting from me this month. It was paid. Just ask the power company.

With growing dread, I called the power company. This conversation started out with a bit of negotiation, since the bill was in her name and not mine, but it was unquestionably my debit card that had paid it for months and months, and they had the account marked as a secondary trailer brought in on a farm. They could tell from the address and my own much longer-standing account that it was on my property. Finally, the supervisor confirmed to me that no, no payment had been made that month yet for Mom's power bill.

I reported this back to Mom, who immediately concluded that the receptionist had stolen it. So sneaky and deceptive, sitting there acting innocent, telling Mom no receipt was required. All the time, she had been planning to steal that cash. In fact, now that Mom thought about it, her eyes had been shifty and her attitude not quite straightforward. Mom was absolutely convinced she had been robbed.

I sent off a mass prayer request email to the family and the pastor asking for urgent attention to this matter. I could already tell that this situation was rapidly exploding. I also kept trying to talk to Mom. I know that logic isn't advertised as the best approach for people with dementia, but Mom was never typical in anything in her life. Reasoning actually *did* work with her pretty well sometimes, even well beyond 2008, even into her quite advanced illness years. At other times, it would fall flat, but she responded to it much more often than she was "supposed" to, sometimes even when other more recommended approaches failed. She had had such a scientific mind in her competent life, I think, that like her advanced vocabulary, that lasted long past the markers where most others with dementia start to lose touch with it. Therefore, I kept analysis as one of several strategies to try with her in her illness. It wasn't always or even usually the first one, but it was there in the bag.

With this situation, I knew she had been worried about the winter power bill; it would make perfect sense that that was pressing on her mind and that she might dream it. She had vivid dreams all her life. I tried gently approaching it from this direction. No, she insisted. It was true. The facts here were that the power company employed thieves, and they had taken her money. I was calling her a liar.

Efforts to clarify that I wasn't calling her a liar, simply thought she might be dreaming or mistaken, yielded nothing. She continued to insist that the bill was paid and that furthermore, she was going to double-check that I didn't pay it again. I agreed to check everything out and promised to ask Vicki, still routinely in touch with the Arkansas family, if this relative or anyone else had been in the state lately.

Then I received a call back from the supervisor at the power company, the same woman I had wound up talking to when I was trying to determine whether a payment had been made on Mom's account. She said that Mom had called up there herself, accused the receptionist of theft, and wanted her fired. In fact, Mom also wanted to file police charges.

Backed into this corner, there was only one thing I could do. The poor receptionist couldn't lose her job over this. I told the supervisor that Mom had dementia, was apparently slipping into full-blown delusions, and that I was positive all this had never happened. The supervisor recorded that statement. She said that from her own conversation with Mom, Mom had not sounded rational or competent at all. I apologized for everything. She sympathized but pointed out that this was a serious charge. I acknowledged that and said that we would take further steps on our end to try to manage things better. If any trouble with the police came up, I told her to just refer them to me, and I would give them the same statement. I was certain that no theft ever had taken place.

The supervisor did tell me that she was marking on Mom's account that I was authorized to discuss its details. On any future call, anyone there would be glad to speak to me without the extensive discussion required that first time. Obviously, none of them ever wanted to speak to Mom again.

I then gently attempted to tell Mom that trying to lose people's jobs for them and talking about police charges was premature. We were still gathering details on what had happened, waiting for Vicki's report from Arkansas, and such. Let's get all the facts in first. She blew up. Not only was I calling her a liar to her face, but now I had called her a liar to other people. She launched into a tirade about my ethics and how far I had fallen from my raising. Diabolical was one word that came up.

The words hurt, but they weren't the worst of it. I knew that it was the disease talking, that she in her right mind didn't think that of me. What hurt and even scared me more was the situation itself. This was ominous.

In retrospect, it seems that I should have realized it before, given her ample imagination, her forceful personality, and her propensity toward slaying lizards, but this was the first time that I clearly saw some of those future mile markers. Memory loss was not going to be the hardest element of her illness to deal with. We would not have a slow spiral down into mental fog. There would be hallucinations, delusions. There probably would be even violence. Looking at it objectively, I had to admit she was capable of fighting, up to and including physically, if she felt threatened. She would push back against the expanding mental shadows. She would battle vigorously, even if futilely. Mom, who always could make even trivial things a campaign, was now in a struggle for control of her mind, her lifelong worst fear, and she would throw every ounce she could into that war. As bad as things suddenly were, they were going to get worse.

And nothing at all I could do would help that.

That Sunday, two days after the crisis began, came another Singers concert. Mom did not want to attend either church that morning or the concert in the afternoon. She had missed church far more often than she had gone recently, citing her legs and the winter, but that day, she wasn't speaking to me, though she was in fact saying plenty.

In the worst timing imaginable, I also had a lunch date that Sunday to be introduced to a man I'd never met before. Some members at church who were trying to set me up with a friend of theirs took us both out to lunch after service. Nobody at the table except me had any idea what was going on that weekend. Mom even had been included originally in the invitation, and they hadn't realized the extent of her problems when they asked. They did not know her closely, and her illness had not yet advanced to the stage of having updates in the church prayer reminder.

(The fact that church members trying to set me up on a date would include my mother in the invitation for the first group meeting illustrates perfectly how close the two of us were and how much the entire church knew that fact. We were always side by side at church, had been during our entire membership there of well over a decade, even when we weren't living together. I indeed wouldn't have minded a bit had Mom, in anything resembling her right mind, been with us at that lunch.)

The man was very nice, a good Christian, and had a reserve that appealed to me. I've never appreciated the Golden Retriever style approach from men or even people in general, and unfortunately, several men who had wished to date me seemed to specialize in it. With this man, we did wind up subsequently going out for a few months, and we got along well enough, but the spark, the chemistry was missing. I don't think that was because of the crisis with Mom, but undoubtedly, her situation often demanded priority of my energy during our entire acquaintance, and it definitely didn't help my dating life much. I did, of course, tell him within a few weeks that my mother had dementia and was getting worse, and he sympathized.

After that lunch, I went on to make call time for the afternoon's concert. We were singing a Bach cantata, but as we warmed up and made our final preparation, the empty hall loomed out beyond the platform and kept drawing my eye. That weekend, I knew that it was over, that the concert back in early December had been Mom's last time ever hearing this group that she had loved so much. I found another song we had sung a few years earlier running through my mind, a poignant Civil War ballad telling of a family's gathering after losing one of their own: "We shall meet, but we shall miss him. There will be one vacant chair."[17]

That was in warm-up. During the concert itself, Bach took hold of me. I was glad that it was Bach that day, for I sorely needed it. If Rachmaninoff is the perfect expression of moods and undercurrents surging along, hitting occasional rapids, and ultimately resolving into harmony at the end, Bach is the perfect expression of unshakeable order. Bach above all makes sense. Every single note is placed in almost mathematical precision, and each work proclaims beginning to end that there is structure, there is resolution, things will all come out as they should. Even in fugal portions, the cosmos, the overall plan, never wavers. Rachmaninoff is marvelous when you want to process feelings and cast them into harmony. Bach is even better when you simply are too storm blasted to process the feelings anymore.

After the concert, I drove home alone, taking the back and slightly longer way. For the first time in memory, part of me didn't want to return home to Erdenheim. The Bach had calmed the storm enough that I could resume praying about it to more extent than just, "Lord, help!" The entire drive back was a prayer; I never even turned on the radio or a CD. That drive home from that concert was my Gethsemane of Mom's illness. I prayed for this cup to pass, for escape not for me but for her, that somehow this road I now saw so clearly outlined ahead could be avoided, even if by her premature death. No instant answer appeared, no miracle handed down from heaven, yet I felt the presence and comfort of God more strongly with each mile. Whatever was ahead, it was in his hands, not mine, and I gradually was reminded that his were big enough to hold even this.

"If I forget, yet God remembers."

Back at the farm, the power company saga showed no signs of losing voltage. I had tried several times from that first day on to tell Mom that I was dealing with the situation myself, that it was being taken care of, and she didn't need to worry about it anymore, but she didn't trust me on this. My statement to the supervisor that first afternoon contradicting her story had shattered any credibility I had with Mom in this whole episode. Still, I couldn't let the employee suffer job or legal consequences. After Mom had escalated publicly to the threat of police action, I had had no choice then but to refute her equally publicly.

A second version of her story now appeared. Once in a while, it was no longer the receptionist to whom she had given the cash with no receipt. No, a woman had been sitting in the lobby waiting who said she was looking for a job there, and Mom had given the money to her to pay the bill. But most of the time, the target remained the receptionist, who had flat out stolen it and ought therefore to be fired and charged for the theft.

Vicki heard back from her contacts in Arkansas. As expected, nobody from that branch of the family had been anywhere near our state recently. Mom, when presented with this fact, said that the man who had come was from the estranged branch, so of course, he wouldn't admit anything to the remainder of the family, and they wouldn't have known he was out of town for a few days. There really was a branch of the family that had had some tension with the rest, the cold ashes of an old blazing dispute decades earlier over my great-grandparents' will. But this was hardly at the level of the Hatfields and the McCoys, and there was no reason to deny something so simple. Again, this man had never been close to Mom and hadn't seen her in forever. For her to be the one person locally he tried to see if he wanted to visit the state and renew acquaintances was unrealistic. If he were around these parts, he would have looked up Vicki, known to be in touch with the family all along and far easier to find.

On top of everything, I actually did, of course, pay her power bill. This set off a new tirade. I gladly would have tried to conceal that from her, but she asked me directly, in full righteous indignation, and insisted on a yes/no answer, refusing to accept generalizations that everything had been taken care of. "I *knew* you were going to do that. You just gave those *thieves* double money, and I didn't have any to spare." Then once again, she would ask for a ride to the police station to file charges.

Ultimately, I realized that nothing short of digging my own heels in was going to work here. I finally told Mom that no matter what, she was not going to be allowed to create difficulties for that receptionist either at her job or with the law. Whomever she spoke to, I promptly would counter her story. My popularity subsequently took even more of a nosedive, but Mom knew that I meant it, and, hurt and angry, she backed off and let consequences for the "theft" go.

She didn't forget my statement, either, though I was prepared to repeat it as often as necessary if she did. After that, the receptionist permanently vanished from her target sights, but from this point on, I would continue to drift in and out of them in my now alternating personalities of good and evil daughter. I was more often good than evil to her, but the days of accusation still hurt when they came, even knowing that it was the disease talking. Never before February 22 had I expected her to turn against me. I probably should have anticipated that it might happen, but I did not. Not between us.

Even more painful was that I hadn't grasped until then the full scope of her course, where we were heading, and my helplessness to make some situations easier for her. Prior to the power company fiasco, I had thought of dementia as primarily a disease of memory; now I saw that that was just one part of it. Also, my help ultimately was not going to be enough for Mom, and while I had known that on some level as book knowledge, the powerlessness hadn't fully seized me with cold certainty before. The one aspect that made February harder for me than the truly awful summer that followed is that in February, I was blindsided. I was left scrambling, trying to figure out how possibly to make the situation easier for her and calm her down (while avoiding police charges), and failing at every turn. By the summer of 2008, I had no expectations left and was just taking it moment by moment, trying my best to be there for her in each one.

For her, of course, the shock had to be even greater. She wasn't able to put it in the framework of the illness for explanation; to her, I truly had started calling her a liar, not only privately but to others. Many were the hours that I lay awake at night with my heart breaking for her and praying that somehow, she would find some peace, not just ultimately in heaven but here on earth as she went through her greatest fear.

Even after Mom gave up her plots for justice for the power company, I knew I had to get medical documentation for the course ahead. Mom was vehemently anti-doctor and hadn't seen one in years, but we had to get an official diagnosis, and I needed an expert opinion written down to help the next time she tried to file charges on someone or something similar. Also, she probably wasn't going to be safe living at Erdenheim indefinitely, though I would keep her here as long as possible, and I realized now that I couldn't necessarily count on her cooperation if she ever needed to be placed in a care facility.

Two-by-Twice had had a small account for a few years from a neuropsychologist. This doctor had sent extensive competency testing results to be transcribed, several pages per patient, and Mom, the psychology major, had handled that typing. She had found it fascinating and always enjoyed working on that account, even wishing there were more of it. She also had her soft heart touched by many of the patient histories, especially as she was dealing with her parents' illness at the same time. More than once over the years, well before her own fall, I found Mom sitting at her computer praying instead of typing. "I have to pray for this one and his family," she would tell me. "I can at least do that much."

Seeing a possible opening here with the past relationship with that neuropsychologist, I made Mom a proposal. She was already familiar with this doctor and with the competency screenings. If she would submit to one of those full testing sessions, just like the ones she had typed, and the results proved officially that there was nothing at all wrong with her, I would accept that, apologize, and never bring up the subject or challenge her mentally again. In short, this was her golden opportunity to prove me wrong.

Mom eagerly accepted that deal with one further condition. She wanted me to get tested, too, as she had concluded that my irrationality in the last week was so overboard that obviously *I* was the one developing dementia.

The mental dollar signs were already spinning in my mind; I knew that this testing had run to a few thousand back years earlier when Granddaddy had had it done. Mom had been most relieved at that time that Medicare had covered it. But Mom wasn't yet sixty-five. There was no Medicare, no insurance of any kind. To get this done, it would have to be on a cash basis. I had just borrowed some money back in January from a good friend for further improvements on Mom's trailer; I hoped she could add another aliquot given this crisis. But something, somehow, had to be done.

To avoid the cost of two full screenings, I agreed that if Mom went first and passed with flying colors, as she was certain she would, I would get screened myself after that. She accepted this bargain, and I called the neuropsychologist.

The doctor was quite sympathetic on the phone. I reported a thumbnail version of the power company drama, and she agreed that we needed official documentation urgently. She did politely bring up the issue of cost, and I assured her that she would be paid. She even had an unexpected opening within the next week from a cancellation, and she offered me that appointment.

The day of the testing, Mom was as painstakingly prepared as if going to church on Easter Sunday. Her hair was immaculate, her makeup pristine, her dress perfect. She was the walking image of someone with her act together. To her mind, she was attending her justification, and on the way there, she made sure to remind me of my end of the bargain. Once it was established that she wasn't having any problems, I had to get evaluated myself. I agreed.

Both of us were present during the initial interview, and the power company tale was relived in detail. Mom got riled up just repeating it, and the doctor had to remind her to calm down. Mom's speech was still fluent, her conversational ability still high, but skillful questioning pulled out the facts that she couldn't remember what she had done the last weekend, couldn't remember the menu of her most recent meal, and had stopped driving. She blamed this again on Morgan but grudgingly admitted after that that she had gotten lost a few times. She did state that nobody in the family besides me had any concern over her or had ever doubted her ability to function.

After about forty-five minutes, the doctor kicked me out. The actual testing would be done privately. I had brought a book, but I spent more time in the lobby praying than reading. The whole process took hours.

At one point, Mom came out for a bathroom break, and while she was in there, the doctor came over to me and simply said, "I'm sorry." The tests weren't even completed, much less scored, but the verdict was already there in her tone, not that I had doubted it. Unless I myself was going crazy, Mom was in full-blown dementia now. I did take the opportunity to tell the doctor that other family members definitely were worried about her and also had noticed issues even long distance.

Mom rejoined us, and then the testing resumed. Finally, approaching 5:00, they emerged, and Mom turned the wrong way when heading for the bathroom again before leaving, giving a live demonstration of her ability to get lost in a building these days.

Scoring would take another several hours, and the doctor gave us an appointment for the next week to receive results. As I drove away, Mom said, with her chin up, "Well, I'm glad we got that over with." I asked her what she had thought of the testing, and she said it had been fun. "It's not like it was challenging or anything." Sitting there in her Sunday best, the outer display fiercely trying to hide the inner decline, she chatted about Erdenheim on the way home—until she fell asleep.

The results the next week confirmed that decline and even spelled it out further than expected. Mom was so good, incredibly good, at keeping a front. Her verbal IQ was still in the ninety-fifth percentile scored against others her age, but the overall performance IQ hit the fourteenth percentile. The doctor commented that it was unusual to have verbal ability still that high with such blatant functional deficits. "Her brain is failing asymmetrically." When the doctor said that, it reminded me of Mom over and over again through the years pulling out a favorite phrase: "Why be normal?"

On the individual tests of different areas of memory and functioning, her scores were abysmal, her best being thirtieth percentile and most of them falling below the first. Her worst recorded score was in the 0.02nd percentile, and there was one test on which she did even worse than that, as she totally stalled on it and could not complete that test even with cues.

The doctor related it all objectively, going into each test, and Mom sat there and absorbed it quietly. Like Granddaddy years earlier, she didn't challenge the results (not right then, anyway). The doctor concluded with her extremely strong recommendations to see a medical doctor for a full physical, see a lawyer ASAP, and listen to her family, who did have her best interests at heart. She did say that in her opinion, Mom was still capable of understanding and signing legal documents on a good day, but that the time window for that was rapidly closing.

The diagnosis was dementia, probably Alzheimer's type, though the doctor did confirm that Mom was young to be so advanced in it. Mom was very quiet upon leaving. That evening at home, she bravely composed a group email to the family in which she admitted the results of the screening.

The next day, I called both a doctor and a lawyer. I was afraid that Mom's compliance would be only temporary; she probably would start to manufacture reasons why the testing was invalid. Having belatedly realized that she was going to fight this disease with every ounce of the formidable mental energy she possessed,

I doubted she would surrender after just one battle. I had to secure legal paperwork as soon as possible, as well as a doctor's appointment. I thought Mom might reverse her decision on seeing the doctor in particular; she had given so many excuses for years on why she didn't need physicians.

Unfortunately, when I called her internist (she did have one, just hadn't seen him in years), he had moved away. The large clinic where he had practiced referred me to another of their partners, and the doctor accepting new patients had no openings for an initial appointment until September. It was now the beginning of March. I doubted that I could get her in faster anywhere else, so I took that appointment and prayed that she still would be willing to keep it.

The lawyer was much more expedient. I called a lawyer in the church, one who had known Mom for over fifteen years, and explained the situation. He was brisk, efficient, and helpful. "I know exactly what you need, and I'll write it up." He did say that Mom would have to sign papers voluntarily, and I said she probably would (at that moment, but please, hurry, before she got riled up over the phone company or someplace else and I became the diabolical daughter again). He promised swift action, and we made an appointment a few days later at his office to sign.

Mom was still cooperative on that day, and we sat together in his office as he produced a power of attorney that was many pages long and apparently included everything but the kitchen sink. I would be grateful over and over again in the coming years for his care in drawing up that document. With one exception—more on that later—it was accepted by every person or entity

I ever had to deal with regarding Mom, clear down to the medical university to which her body was donated after her death.

He carefully explained to Mom that this would give me full power to act on her behalf. She agreed that this was a good idea "in case something happens." Then came the signing. He had three copies to be signed, to yield three originals, and as he handed her a pen, he said, "Of course, you know what today's date is."

I couldn't help stiffening up in dismay. I was certain that Mom did not know the date. She was awful on dates and days of the week anymore. Sure enough, she promptly looked over at me and asked. I told her, and she signed as the lawyer frowned. "You aren't supposed to cue her," he admonished.

Mom moved on to the second copy and there, mere seconds after signing the first, couldn't remember the date. She again asked me, and that time, I was meekly silent. She then asked the lawyer. After a moment, he started holding up fingers, and she read the digits off easily and dated the document.

On to the third copy, where for the third time within the last minute, she drew a complete blank at the date. She once more asked me, then asked him. The lawyer looked at me, a silent communication. *This is pushing it*. I'm grateful that he had known Mom and me for years already. She in fact wasn't unwilling to sign. I do think she understood that day what she was signing, and he knew that I wasn't trying to take advantage of her. Finally, he simply told her the date, and Mom filled it in for the third time.

We thanked him and left with several copies as well as originals. As we exited the office, she smiled at me and said, "This was a good idea, Deb. Life is uncertain."

Yes. Life is uncertain. I walked beside her at her snail's pace to the car with the official, legal, invaluable paperwork in my hand, wishing with all my heart that I would never have to use it and knowing even in the wish that I would.

# 8.

# *The Bad Summer*

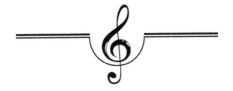

As I had feared, Mom's acceptance of her diagnosis was short lived. The first effort at denial came when she called me one day and told me that she had forgotten to inform the neuropsychologist about her head injury on her tenth birthday in the bicycle accident. Therefore, with the doctor not taking this into account in scoring all of the tests, the results were skewed. She didn't have Alzheimer's after all, just some stable long-term residuals of the old head injury.

In the first place, Mom had told the doctor about that bike accident. During the initial interview, which I sat in on, the doctor had been very thorough in extracting any sort of medical history, including asking about injuries at any point in life. The bike wreck was actually referred to in the summary report in the history section. Beyond that, of course, there was no way that a head injury over fifty years previously could make someone score in the 0.02nd percentile on functionality tests when that person had been a working, fully productive member of society for decades in the meantime.

I showed Mom that line in the medical history in the report. She conceded that the doctor had had the information about the wreck but still insisted that she hadn't applied it in scoring the tests. I let it go, but the sinking feeling in the pit of my stomach dating from the power company episode remained. Memory loss wasn't going to be the hardest symptom of the illness. Mom was going to fight her lifelong worst fear, losing control of her mind, with all the considerable energy she could throw at it.

Later on, a second explanation for the test results emerged. She decided that she had had Alzheimer's, a very mild case, but had cured it with vitamins and supplements and was quite healthy again mentally.

That spring, I quit my part-time job as a home health aide. I absolutely loved the work, but it took me away from home far too much, and with the situation imploding, I wanted to be there as much as possible. The transcription I could do at the farm over the computer, though as 2008 progressed, it became by far the year of lowest production I'd ever hit on typing. Stressors and interruptions with Mom avalanched. Work knew what was going on, and bless them, they cut me ample slack. It didn't pay the bills, but at least I didn't lose my job.

Michael and James both came to visit that spring, Michael for a few days at Easter, James a month or two later. Michael hadn't seen Mom since his wedding back in 2005, and he was shocked. Mom's physical decline alone over that period was incredible. Her walking was tentative and at snail's speed, even using a cane; I timed her once in late summer 2008 out in the yard at two feet a minute. The mental failure was less visible but equally obvious when you spent extended time with her.

Easter. The season of life, of promise. That Easter, I went alone to church in Springfield, having musical obligations there. I took Kipling, the little Focus I had bought back in January for better fuel efficiency on the aide work, not knowing then about Mom's imminent mental crash and how short lived that job would be. Michael, staying back at the farm, borrowed Coleridge and drove Mom down to a little country church nearby for Easter services.

On my solo drive into the city, I thought of the past two Easters and how quickly life could change. Easter 2006 was when the nursing home had notified us that they thought Granddaddy was entering his last days. Mom and I went to church together, but after the service, she had driven on down to the nursing home in Morgan to see him.

On Easter 2007, it was nineteen degrees. Bright and sunny but nineteen degrees! Mom's memory problems were advancing but still were simply memory problems. She and I went together in Coleridge to church, and the congregation still held our sunrise service outside, though I remember everybody packed down the hall inside the doors, waiting for the start signal. Nobody went out early to get a seat. When the pastor gave the word, we all spilled out to the chairs on the lawn, and everyone shivered through a brilliant sunrise. Mom said she was having a little aching in her legs from the cold, but the effect on her walking wasn't that noticeable yet. Her primary concern that morning was for *me*, for my knee that I've had three surgeries on. It hated cold weather and indeed objected to that cold morning. But Mom, sitting outside in nineteen degrees for over half an hour, handled it fine and walked steadily back inside once the service concluded. She then headed down the stairs to fellowship hall for breakfast and later back up more stairs for Sunday School and choir.

Now, Easter 2008, only one year later, Mom could barely walk, and we had delusions, hallucinations, and paranoia added into the mix, with violence, I feared, potentially lurking just around the corner. The year loomed ahead of me, and I had no idea how long she would be able to be kept safely at home. The services that morning were especially poignant to me. Life. Hope. Promise after darkness. Even in years like 2008, which would only head downhill from February, He is risen indeed.

James came with his wife, Beth, in late spring, bringing a small air conditioner for Mom's trailer. Mom enjoyed the visit, but conversation with her by that point was like hearing bells tolling in the distance announcing a funeral. More and more, even in the memories, she started inserting threats and helplessness that had never been there in the first place. I remember during James and Beth's short stay that we were all talking in the living room of Mom's trailer one night, and she launched into the story of the house fire. I had progressively become younger with each telling, and by now, I was a baby in her arms. She told of standing outside the house holding me and feeling absolutely helpless to do anything, unable to stop the unfolding disaster. She was literally in tears as she described her utter powerlessness and that all she could do was hold the baby. Gone was her actual brisk efficiency that night, calling the fire department and then trying to save a few pieces from the house once we kids were safely out. James, Beth, Daniel, and I just looked at one another.

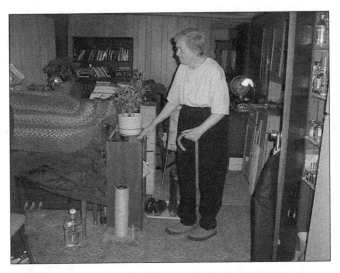

**Mom in her trailer at the farm in 2008.**

The summer of 2008 was almost indescribable. Fear and threat were the overarching themes. Most of the books and articles on dementia suggest not attempting to reorient a patient to reality, simply letting them inhabit their confused world if that's what they are fixed into. Mom's delusions, however, made this course impossible. Nothing was pleasantly confused memories of the past or of doing former jobs again. No, with her, there was constant threat of attack. You can't calm someone down by confirming their belief that the place is on fire or that stalkers are outside attempting to abduct us. Nor would she ever accept attempted reassurance that the situation was being dealt with by others and that she didn't have to worry. She needed to respond to the threat herself.

Fire was one of her major fixations. I heard the old story several times a week, growing each time in terror, and now new mental fires started to ignite. Mom had always been extremely fire conscious. A few times since she'd gotten the trailer, she had worried about it catching on fire, and I had reminded her of that several-thousand-dollar electrical upgrade by the master electrician, which would reassure her.

In 2008, however, she started smelling and later even occasionally seeing fires. I would be typing at my place, and the phone would ring with Mom in a panic. "I smell smoke!" I'd drop work and go tearing over, and there was nothing. I would walk around the trailer, calm her, and finally return to my house. Often, only five minutes later, another call would come, and we would be back to square one with no memory of the previous call. Later, when she would actually see a flame flicker in a corner, it got even worse. Trying to reassure someone there is no fire when they swear they smelled or saw one is an exercise in worried helplessness. Doing it multiple times a week wears on you. Still, I often thought that as bad as that summer was for me, it must have been far worse for Mom, living in terror as the walls of her mind's fort crumbled.

Then there was Frankenfridge. The refrigerator that came with Mom's trailer was an older model but seemed to work fine. Mom, however, worried about it at times in those first two years living there. It did feel warm on the side when the motor was running, but it never seemed to me any warmer than other refrigerators would be. She even boycotted it for a while, afraid it would catch on fire, and used a microfridge instead.

In 2008, however, the refrigerator progressed in Mom's mind from simply old and possibly ready for retirement due to aging wiring. It became first acutely dangerous, then by the end of the summer actively plotting. She constantly worried that it would catch on fire (even after it was unplugged and once more boycotted). Ultimately, she began to wonder if *it* was watching *her*. Before long, I took to calling the thing Frankenfridge mentally and in updates to the family, though never to her face. Sometimes, you have to laugh, even when you want to cry.

Frankenfridge left us in late summer. Mom was having trouble sleeping with that refrigerator lurking in the next room, so I listed it on Freecycle. Several people responded promptly, and I took the first family, warning them in advance to discount anything Mom said and promising that there was nothing except possibly age wrong with Frankenfridge. The family arrived in a borrowed pickup to collect it. They were a father, mother, and two children, and they were nearly in tears themselves in gratitude. They had no refrigerator at all, they said. They smiled and thanked us, were nice to Mom, and left with their prize. That particular worry then disappeared, somehow never forwarded to the microfridge, but it had had a lot of company, and the other fixations and delusions were increasing.

Stalkers appeared on the horizon of Mom's mind. She worried that she had heard someone outside, had seen someone slink by a window. People were looking in. She heard laughter. It was always laughter for some reason, never spoken threats but cold laughter, "like in a horror movie, Deb." Sometimes, the prowlers became one specific person from her past (an old boyfriend she'd rejected back in high school). Sometimes, they were just anonymous laughter and faces. As summer wore on, these visitors grew bolder. Now they not only laughed but also pulled her out the windows and sometimes captured her on the porch when she stepped outside. She was able to fight her way free of them each time by her report. She would, in her mental scenarios, bolt back inside (yes, bolt, run, and other high-speed words that she was no longer capable of) and then would promptly report to me her narrow escape.

It was in connection with the prowlers that she started to ask about the gun. I had a gun, and unfortunately, she knew that from before her dementia. In everything, she never forgot that fact. She would call and demand it so she could "defend" herself. I came up with excuses each time, usually that I was working right then (or trying to, at least, though hardly any work got done anymore). I kept hoping that if I put her off, she'd forget about it, but she wanted that gun more and more. I hid it most carefully, but I seriously was starting to worry about the health of innocent UPS or FedEx men who might happen by with a delivery. Fortunately, my house was in front, and you had to pass mine on the driveway to reach hers.

In the days surrounding July 4, she called in an absolute panic because of fireworks. Erdenheim is in deep country. There are always fireworks going off out here close to the Fourth. But Mom was convinced that it was Al Qaeda. She was still voraciously reading her news sites on the computer daily. I told her no, it was only the Fourth of July. "Oh, okay." A few minutes later, she would be beside herself again. "We're under attack!"

Daniel had retreated in her mind all the way back to a napping baby by this point. "Shh!!! Don't wake up Daniel!" I couldn't speak above a whisper in her trailer if his bedroom door was shut. Yes, those conversations when I would try to reassure her that the refrigerator wasn't in fact dangerous, that the place wasn't on fire, and that prowlers weren't surrounding us were conducted in whispers. Even when he wasn't there and was off at work, she would fuss about waking him up. When I would point out that he wasn't even home, that his car was gone, she'd think he was missing, like an infant who had crawled off. When told that he was at work, she would immediately call his work to check. She made multiple calls that summer to the bookstore, where he worked, just to verify his presence. Even the bookstore began to comment on her frequent calls. One day when he had a dentist appointment first and was late getting there, she was completely in a panic because he hadn't arrived yet.

Daniel told me later in September that Mom, until the last month or so, didn't show the delusions and hallucinations in front of him. He saw the memory loss, of course, but he only had my reports on the other symptoms, though he had no reason to doubt the truth of them. That did change starting in August, when she exhibited several openly delusional moments with him.

All summer, I was the one she called with a fire, prowler, Frankenfridge, etc. She wanted me to solve it, to fix the situation. All my life, I've been organized, even over organized. I'm good at putting things in place. Somehow, she held on to recognition of that, I think, and she sometimes wanted me to fix everything that was wrong. This continued on through the nursing home years; she on some days would turn to me for a solution to the unsolvable. I only wish I could have helped her. I did, at least, still seem to be able to calm her down that summer, but it wouldn't last, and five minutes later, here we would go again. Not only my work but also sleep was impacted. She had zero time sense anymore. She would call even with minor things ("don't forget that I need more yogurt next time you go to the store"), and when told it was 3:00 a.m., she would look out the window in surprise at the darkness and say, "Oh, sorry. I hadn't realized."

It was toward the end of that summer that I realized that I was actively wishing her to die, for release for her sake more than mine. Each morning, I would go over to her trailer to feed barn cats, something she wasn't capable of doing anymore, but she worried that they weren't getting fed unless she saw me physically get the food and take it out to them. That belief was easy enough to accommodate, not being threatening or unsafe. I simply kept the barn cat food in her place and came in every morning to dish up, then took it back out to distribute it. Every morning, I opened the trailer door, and my first look was to the right, to her bedroom door and her bed immediately beyond. I could see her in bed from the door, and I would watch to see if she was breathing. Once I realized what I was thinking and even wishing daily as I took that first look, I felt guilty about that for a while. Then I considered it and decided there was nothing to feel guilty about. I was under incredible stress, she was under even more, and thoughts like that were going to crop up at times. It was an understandable human reaction to the situation. Besides, it would, in fact, be a step up for her, if that were God's timing, of course.

There were two symptoms that never emerged even in that worst time. The first was wandering. Mom never left Erdenheim, never even tried. She didn't even leave mentally; there was no retreat in her mind to homes of yesteryear. No, she knew she was at the farm, and that still was where she wanted to be. Later on, she would try to escape from the nursing home, but not once while on Erdenheim did she attempt to leave or even unintentionally wander away in confusion. She did love that farm, our earthly home that we had dreamed of together for years even before the reality.

The second symptom she lacked was that her language never slipped. I have heard that many demented people use profanity at times even if they never had in their lives before. Mom didn't. That would hold true until her death, even through the nursing home years. She remained in that aspect the preacher's kid raised by Granddaddy, whose worst word I ever heard, including from his demented years, was "fiddlesticks," and by Grandmother, who I'm sure literally would have washed a child's mouth out with soap. Even in the bad summer, I would notice this with Mom at times and remember the piano recital ("Fish Feathers!") and smile.

Of course, there were other days, good days, even that summer. They grew much rarer, but they still occurred. Not every moment had a fire or prowlers or Al Qaeda or Frankenfridge. Sometimes when I was mowing the grass, I would set up a chair outside, and she would sit there and watch me and pet cats. Mom always looked so at home with a cat in her lap; you could almost hear her purring along with the feline.

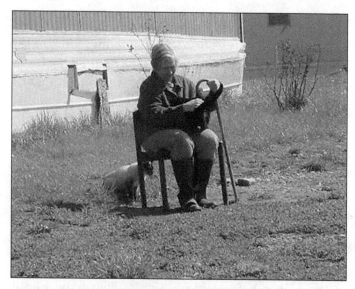

**Mom petting cats at Erdenheim.**

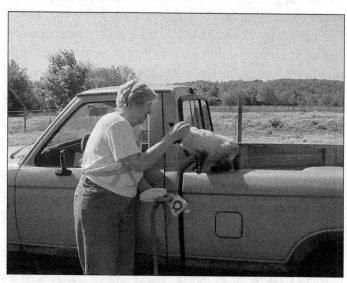

**Mom, Chiaroscuro, and Morgan, who was just a yard ornament by this stage.**

She still talked about the flowers and landscaping she wanted to do. We still could discuss books, and her favorite poem remained Theodore Tilton's "Even This Shall Pass Away."

It was on July 12, not long after the Al Qaeda fears, that I received an email from her that I kept carefully on file. I have it to this day. I would read it over during bad days and remind myself again that even the disease was temporary. There is hope; there is promise. God can handle it. Ultimately, there is healing. The email quoted a hymn by Mary Lathbury (Mom still knew every song in the hymnal by memory then) with Mom's own tag line P.S.

Sent: *July 12, 2008 06:27*
Subject: *Evening at Erdenheim*

*"Day is dying in the west;*
*Heaven is touching earth with rest.*
*Wait and worship while the night*
*Sets her evening lamps alight*
*Through all the sky.*

*Holy, holy, holy, Lord God of Hosts.*
*Heaven and earth are full of Thee;*
*Heaven and earth are praising Thee,*
*O Lord, most high!"*[18]

*Erdenheim: The most peaceful spot on earth.*

*Mom*

# 9.

# *Limits*

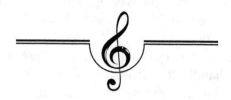

I had nothing left.

By the end of the summer of 2008, the situation was getting truly unsafe. Mom's world was filled with prowlers, Al Qaeda, fires, and even wild animals now stalking around her trailer and lying in wait for her on the porch. She reported having to fight her way past them when she went outside. Sometimes she was even pulled out through the windows when she was inside.

Her obsession with getting the gun was increasing, and she had even mentioned testing her knives and noticing that not one of them was very sharp. (That much was true. Mom deliberately never kept sharp knives throughout her life. She was never into cooking to the point where a sharp one would be needed in food preparation, and our family could cut ourselves with a butter knife, much less anything more lethal. "We get our grace at the cross," she would say often. "We certainly don't have any otherwise.")

In late summer, in the midst of the worst period of hallucinatory fires, Mom actually did leave the stove on once. It was only once that I was aware of, though she might have done it more often and concealed that after she noticed later. On that one day, I came in and found the burner on full with nothing there. Oddly, as paranoid and hysterical as she could get with imaginary fires, she was unruffled by this actual threat and dismissed the lapse. "Oh, nothing was on it. It's not that big a deal. Everybody does that now and then."

She also had started falling. Her balance and use of her legs had continued to plummet, and a friend had donated a walker. I was a little worried that Mom would be insulted by this gift and stick stubbornly to her cane, but she appreciated it and did start using it— after a fashion. Sometimes, she would be between the walker arms in the correct position. At other times, she would push the walker in front of her with it either backwards or even sideways, pushing on an arm bar. Even accepting the walker, she sometimes forgot it and wandered off unassisted to another room. She fell several times in that last month and once couldn't get up on her own. She did call me then, and as when she left the stove on, she was completely nonchalant. Not a big deal, just needed a little help getting up, but things like that were bound to happen when you got older.

In short, she was no longer safe out at the farm, and I wasn't convinced that the rest of the world was, either. I do think she would have been capable of attacking a UPS man or another innocent visitor thinking he was a threat. She did later, in the nursing home, exhibit violence.

I was also exhausted. Work was next to impossible, even doing it from home, due to the constant interruptions to help or keep tabs on her. Sleep was also next to impossible for the same reasons. By the beginning of September, I had to admit that if things went on much longer like this, I would break my own health as well as lose my job.

Above all, I had to admit that it wasn't enough. The home provided there at Erdenheim and the supervision that I (full time) and that Daniel (when he wasn't at work) could give simply were no longer enough to keep her or others safe. That was a hard wall to run into for someone who was by personality a fixer, a sorter. I didn't quite take it to Mom's level of slaying mere lizards, but I had always appreciated a good dragon now and then. I had taken pride in solving problems from childhood on. Now, I had to admit that everything I could give her, even if I broke myself on it, was inadequate. I had hit the limit.

Mom still had the doctor's appointment in mid-September with the new internist, the appointment that the neuropsychologist back in March had talked her into scheduling. Realizing that she would have to be placed, I thought back to how this step had been accomplished with Grandmother and Granddaddy. Of course, Mom had been the point person then, and I didn't know all the details, just what she had relayed, but I did remember that their doctors were cooperating and on board with this and had helped smooth the process. So I decided that at that appointment, I would enlist the doctor to start the wheels rolling to get her placed.

As for the facility, there was no question where she would go. The one Mom herself had picked for her own parents after several weeks of comparing was the only choice. Not only did I know firsthand from observation that it was excellent, but Mom was familiar with it already. She had visited there to see her parents for years. I thought the known environment might make the transition easier for her. It would be a long drive for me, but that was way down the list of considerations. Better to have a longer drive for a superior facility. The staff at that one was excellent, and again, many of them already knew Mom. That nursing home had floor staff, not just administration, who had been there for twenty years.

So I mailed the doctor a letter summarizing the situation and a copy of the neuropsych report and cognitive testing, along with the POA, and I contacted the family. Of course, they had been kept updated all the way. I was the front lines throughout Mom's illness, but I bent over backwards to keep everyone in the loop, and the updates increased in frequency as she got worse. From late that summer through the end of her life eight years later, everyone in the direct family would receive an update on Mom at least weekly, more often when things were agitated.

This time, though, I had a specific request. There was that full cognitive testing report, but I also wanted written statements from the others to take to the doctor, further proof for her that I wasn't imagining the issues and going crazy myself. So I asked the family to reply by email, stating their own observations of Mom and her illness and whether they agreed with the decision to seek placement, and I would print those replies off for the doctor.

Everyone responded. The replies varied from Vicki's poignantly brief, "Sadly, I agree," to James, who provided the longest. He gave a nicely detailed timeline of things he and Beth had noticed on visits; they had first seen deficits at Christmas 2002. Daniel responded stating that he had seen only the memory loss himself until the last month, but that now he, too, had witnessed Mom exhibiting blatant delusions in front of him, and he agreed that she was acutely unstable mentally and unsafe. Michael's answer focused more on the physical, but he reported he had been shocked at her decline when he had seen her at Easter and thought even then that she was unsafe living at the farm. Rena's reply not only concurred with Mom's status but contained a line that was balm for me to apply to the nagging sense of failure: "You have gone well beyond your capabilities here."

No one disagreed. The stage was set for that doctor's appointment to start placement proceedings. Mom herself, as of yet, did not know my intentions; I deliberately put that off because I knew that it would throw gasoline on the fire of all her paranoia and suspicions, and I was afraid she would refuse to go to the doctor's appointment. In the end, though, I simply could not blindside her with that plan right there in the office in front of the physician. In the car on the drive to the appointment, I told her that she was going to be placed and that I planned to enlist the doctor's help in getting the ball rolling.

She was in one of her trying-to-be-logical moods, those moods that still could pop out at times long after she was supposed to be past that ability. I gave her as the first reason that she was a safety risk, that I was worried about her at the farm, and I specifically mentioned the ongoing falls. She responded that she was careful, that she knew she had fallen once (it was far more than that), but that she would take care from now on so she wasn't going to fall again. She recited a quite-good list of steps she could take to decrease the possibility. If falls had indeed been the major problem, her well-presented strategy might indeed have helped with that. I next pointed out all her walking difficulty and that it wasn't much of a life basically confined to her trailer at this point. She countered that she loved Erdenheim and had no complaints. Finally, reluctantly, I brought up the dementia. She pulled out the familiar argument that she had formerly had "very mild" Alzheimer's but had cured it with vitamins. This discussion lasted us the last few miles, going in circles, getting nowhere.

When we arrived at the medical office building, I retrieved the wheelchair from the trunk. I had borrowed this wheelchair just a few days ago from a friend at church whose recently deceased father had used it. Mom walking across that parking lot or even dropped off at the door and simply walking across the lobby would have taken half the morning with the walker, and the building was several floors high and sprawling. She had agreed to the temporary use of the wheelchair for this day, and the novelty of getting into that seemed to knock the previous discussion clear out of her mind. After we rolled across the lot to the building and checked in, she chitchatted about cats and flowers, not in a "changing the subject" manner but as if this really were just any routine appointment.

Once we got into the exam room and the doctor entered, I was thrown for a loop myself. The doctor was polite, professional, and clearly had no idea what was going on. Whatever had happened to my letter and testing results mailed the week before, I could tell from her attitude that she had never seen them. A direct question confirmed that, and she asked what the letter had been about. Mom herself was looking at me with genuine confusion and asked the same question. She had indeed forgotten our conversation in the car.

Stuck on the edge of the cliff, I breathed a quick prayer out loud—"Help me, Jesus"—and jumped in full tilt. Mom's expression as I summarized all her increasing problems that year was bewildered beyond disbelief. "Where are you getting all of this?" she asked. "None of that has happened." I offered the doctor the printed-off emails from the family. Mom accused me of making them up.

The doctor stood up, excused herself, and left, taking the emails with her, and Mom and I were alone in the room. She pulled out all the same arguments she had in the car, not realizing the repeat. I was just about in tears myself during this debate, but I never backed away from the decision. Her life at Erdenheim was over. That was a fact, a tragic one but a fact nonetheless.

The doctor opened the door of the room again an eternity of minutes later and asked me to step outside. I did so, leaving Mom to herself. The doctor retreated down to the semiprivacy of the nurses' station and pulled out the envelope with my letter and the test results and POA. She had found it and skimmed it, as well as reading the family emails. She accepted all of that completely, to my relief, and was professionally sympathetic.

The quickest and smoothest way into a nursing home, she said, was to be admitted from an inpatient hospital stay, and she proposed sending Mom to the senior psych unit at the north hospital for a few days, entering through the emergency room so they could check her over physically first. This was on the other side of the city; the medical office building her appointment had been in was next to the south hospital, but there was no psych unit there. The doctor told me that the north hospital social worker could help facilitate placement and would also assist in applying for Medicaid, and further testing could be done on Mom in the meantime. All that sounded good, and the doctor asked if I felt safe driving Mom to the north hospital myself, offering an ambulance if I wished. I replied that I would drive her myself.

So back we both went to the exam room. I don't know exactly what Mom did during that interval alone. Probably she prayed at least part of the time. She had not forgotten what was going on now, but her entire attitude had changed. For the moment, as she had been initially at the results session with the neuropsychologist, she was compliant. All debate had vanished. She said first thing as we entered, "If you want me to go to a nursing home, Deb, I will." I was overwhelmed with gratitude. Even knowing that full cooperation probably wouldn't last many days, I appreciated it, and I still think that part of her deep down did that for me. She saw that I was determined, was not going to yield, but that it was tearing me up to have to do it, and as a gift of love, she gave in for that moment and stopped fighting me directly.

The doctor also was surprised at her abrupt change of heart but seized it. She explained to Mom about the psychiatric admission suggestion prior to facility placement, and Mom agreed without skipping a beat to that as well. The doctor did do a couple of neurological tests on her, the sort that check for strokes, and Mom passed all of those with flying colors. Then she wished us both luck and sent us on our way to the emergency room at the north hospital.

During the drive across the city, Mom remained completely cooperative. She didn't seem confused then; she never lost track of our destination, but she did not argue. I apologized to her for the speed of this and said I really had not planned for an immediate inpatient admission this very day, and she said she believed me. She reiterated that I was a good daughter and also a friend to her. Thank you, Lord, for those moments. Hard enough to do it anyway, infinitely harder to have had to fight her over it.

When we reached the ER at the north hospital, things started to unravel, not with Mom but with the rest of the world. For some reason on this weekday morning, the ER was jam packed, and they were out of rooms. We checked in and were sent to the waiting room, where we sat along with a multitude of others. Time passed. And passed. And passed.

Confusion and hypoglycemia both started to creep in after several hours, the first Mom's, the second mine. I don't technically have diabetes, but all my life, my blood sugar has occasionally just nose-dived, and I do have to keep to a pretty regulated schedule eating, even if I'm not hungry. When we left the farm that morning, I had never expected to be gone this long, and I had nothing with me to eat. The vending machines contained only junk, expensive junk at that. I started feeling increasingly shaky.

Mom, meanwhile, was losing her grasp on the current situation. She wasn't combative, but she had started looking around and asking me, "Tell me why we're here again."

In the middle of that ER waiting room, I suddenly felt as direct a command as if an angel had delivered it personally from heaven. This route might be the easiest way per the doctor, but the Lord wanted me to go back home and call the nursing home myself. We didn't need to wait here any longer.

So we left. First, we went through the McDonald's drive-through. On the way home, I told Mom that I was going to call the nursing home and reiterated that she was going to be placed, just not today. The information was once again new to her, but her compliance held. God had her hand in his that day.

She did make one request, that I not kick Daniel off Erdenheim after she was gone from it herself, and I assured her that I wouldn't. She also had one gut-wrenching realization about halfway home. "My kitty cats!"

I promised her that we would take care of them. Daniel already had said he wanted her current two house cats, and all of the barn cats were being tended by me already. I did say I'd look into feline visits at the nursing home. She had tears in her eyes thinking of a catless residence, but still, she did not fight the placement.

Back home, I got her settled in her trailer, then retreated to my place, spent a minute praying, and called the nursing home. I had no idea to whom I needed to speak, but they quickly got me plugged into their own social worker. She remembered Mom, fortunately. I ran through the current status and admitted up front that there was no funding in place. I would apply for Medicaid, I would apply for anything they suggested, but I was just about at collapse now, and things were unsafe at the farm for her. I needed the most streamlined route to funding and placement possible.

The social worker, bless her, said that they would take Mom at once, fully knowing that the finances were uncertain. They had a female room available, and I could bring Mom down the next day, Tuesday, even with everything else still up in the air.

Thank you, Lord. Thank you. God bless that nursing home. We settled on a time for the next day, early afternoon, and I promised her that I would make the funding search my priority starting Wednesday and that no matter what, they would be paid, somehow, some way, even if it took me years.

I then updated Mom, telling her she would move to the nursing home the next day and again apologizing that I hadn't expected this kind of speed in getting things arranged. I said I'd help her pack in the morning. She was still unresisting.

Next came an update to the family. Much later I did find an email on Mom's computer that she herself had been working on that night. I'm not sure if it was ever sent; it looked like a draft. Even in that, she accepted placement at the moment and was not going to fight me, though she wanted the family to come rescue her and make other arrangements with one of them. She speculated in that update that my motivation for the whole process was wanting to have Erdenheim to myself. Of course, she was perfectly fine herself, so I must have ulterior motives.

But whatever her private thoughts, she did not argue openly with me. From the time when left alone in the doctor's exam room that morning clear through the nursing home the next day, she stopped all active resistance.

The next morning, Tuesday, September 16, 2008, I went over to her trailer to help her pack. In the middle of that process, she threw an independence fit that absolutely cracked me up, not directed at me but at bras. I was going through her drawers, putting her underwear in the luggage, and she straightened up, stuck out that chin in her familiar way, and announced, "I am going to retire from bras. I've decided, and I'm never going to wear one again. I'm now officially retired." That was an easy enough point to concede, and that flare of spirit was so much like Mom.

We included a few houseplants, her CD player and some of her classical music, and her two matching nightstands. At the end, with Kipling packed at her doorstep, I gave her a stuffed cat, one I'd had at my place. Then she said goodbye to her two real cats and thanked them; I nearly lost it watching that.

One still harder moment remained. As we drove around the yard from her trailer back to the driveway to leave, she said, "Goodbye, Erdenheim," and then she tried to launch into the Theodore Tilton poem that was her favorite. "Once in Persia reigned..." She lost it. Groping through the mental fog for lines she had known by heart for decades, she floundered and simply beat out the rhythm. "Dum da dum da dum da dum." The repeated line that concludes every verse finally came back to her. "Even this shall pass away," she said as we turned out of the driveway for her final time.

I had to blink fast to keep seeing the road. I filled in the last verse mentally myself, the one where the king, old and sick, is facing death. The final answer of the poem promises that even death, too, will pass away. And dementia, I added to myself. The disease, the confusion, the loss, the hurt, the misunderstandings, the slow living funeral. Even this shall pass away.

The nursing home was about an hour and a half's drive from the farm, and when we arrived, I retrieved the wheelchair from the trunk once more. The church friend had agreed that we could keep it at the moment. Mom willingly transferred herself out of the car, and we went into the long main hall. An aide had been set as a watch for us, and she greeted us at once and took us back to the social worker's office.

Then came paperwork, of course, a foretaste of what the next few months would hold. The POA was placed in their records. To the question, "Is she competent?", I answered simply, "No." Mom did not object. She seemed very interested in some of the activities described, such as the handicapped-accessible garden and the crafts and music. The only point where she started to get her determination on was when they mentioned the dentist who visited the nursing home. I quickly intervened before she could get rolling on the evil of all dentists and simply said that we declined dental care. The social worker accepted that and noted the chart. Really, I think Mom would have had to be knocked out by that point to submit to a dental exam. I did present for her file that invaluable cognitive testing report, along with all the emails from the family.

Then we were led to her room and met her roommate, a pleasant woman quite a bit younger than Mom but with severe physical, though not mental, problems. She seemed like she would be good company and conversation, and Mom was still very fluent verbally. Mom was already asking her background questions while a staff person and I took a cart out to unload Kipling.

Finally, I left her. I had stayed most of the afternoon, but it was approaching suppertime at the facility, and I needed to find my own meal and drive back to the city. I promised to visit very regularly, and Mom seemed peaceful when I left.

It was Tuesday night, and before returning home, I had Singers. The music was exactly what I needed to conclude that day. Our large work on that current concert cycle was Randall Thompson's "Testament of Freedom," a musical setting of some of the writings of Thomas Jefferson. It was challenging enough to lift me out of the stress of the day momentarily. Even better that night, though, were the other songs we were doing, various folk songs: "Shenandoah," "Down by the Riverside," and "Bound for the Promised Land." The peace and the promise in the music soothed away at least some of the pain.

Then I drove on home alone, back to Erdenheim, which had always been my farm but our joint dream. Now, it was back simply to my farm and dream, and Mom would never return, but I knew that I had had no choice. Everything that I could give her, I had. It simply wasn't enough any longer. I fed the animals, taking a few extra minutes to pet the cats, and then I climbed into bed and fell into the best night's sleep I had enjoyed in months.

# 10.

# *Paperwork*

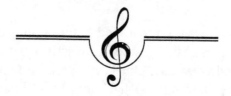

B ack during her working life, Mom had had quite a bit of experience herself with medical paperwork. For decades, she had worked in medical offices, and during her last two jobs before Two-by-Twice, she was office manager. One statistic that she had quoted often to me was her ninety-six percent collection rate during the four years she was office manager at her second-to-last job. (The last job she held too briefly to get valid statistics; that was the one she quit when we started the business.)

Ninety-six percent payment for four years. She was very proud of that figure. Her strategy to achieve it had been simple: with people, she had almost limitless patience. Unless a patient of the clinic totally fell off the radar or unless she diagnosed one with the, to her, cardinal sin of laziness, she never took further steps on their bills, simply sending regular statements and taking without comment whatever they could pay whenever they could pay it. It was extremely rare for her to refer a person to a collection agency.

On the other hand, insurance companies, including Medicare and Medicaid, were treated to Mom in full dragon-slaying armor, girded for battle from the first day of claim. With them, she was utterly relentless. Her firm belief was that most people actually want to pay their bills and will do their best at it as soon as they can, especially if treated with patience, respect, and dignity meanwhile. However, most insurance companies want to dodge paying theirs and actively try to write the checks for as little as possible. Mom also thought the average insurance company was much less efficient than the average patient. Therefore, it was the insurance companies and not the self-pays or uninsureds or remaining-balance individuals who were her focus of tenacious determination.

And it worked. In four years with her at the helm, ninety-six percent of accounts receivable were paid to that office, including both diligently sheep-dogged insurance claims and amounts she patiently waited on from individuals. She relayed to me several tales of grateful patients who paid their accounts once their circumstances improved and who sent the clinic letters thanking her for recognizing them as people going through tough times instead of treating them as deadbeats. Many even said that the clinic was getting paid sooner now that they could, ahead of other creditors who had taken a harder line. (If she ever got any similar letters of appreciation of her tactics from the insurance companies along with their payment for claims, she didn't share those with me.)

I remember spotting a phone number written prominently by her desk when I was in the office one day. Next to it was the acronym SEPM. I inquired, and Mom filled in the letters: Sole Efficient Person at Medicaid. "Took me two years to find one, and the first time I talked to her, I made sure to write her number down. I just call her direct on tough ones now."

Then there was her calendar. She kept a billing calendar, and on claims that were having feet dragged on them, she would schedule a recall to the insurance company. Some were down for every two weeks, some weekly, and if a claim really made Mom's "enough of this nonsense" list, she would call the company daily. "Remember, Deb, bureaucracy respects persistence, even if they keep saying no or making excuses. You are wearing them down."

Another note on that billing calendar showed up every six months: "Resend disability." This related to a patient who was unquestionably disabled and unemployable for medical reasons, with that status permanent. The patient brought the appropriate form from his insurance company to his doctor, and the doctor obligingly filled it out. Mom filed it, and they thought all was well until six months later. At that point, the insurance company asked for another form (the same form, actually, only filled out once again under a new date) to be completed by the office. Mom wrote back objecting and pointing out that they already had the form, and that the patient was *permanently* disabled. That even had been a choice on their own form, with the box "for life" checked in response to the question on anticipated duration. The company replied to Mom, saying, "For the purposes of our company, life is defined as six months. Please refile." Mom responded, saying, "For the purposes of our office, life is defined as life. We will send you another copy of the same original form every six months for your reference." And she did.

In the days after her nursing home placement in 2008, I frequently found myself thinking back to Mom in her bureaucratic paperwork prime, slaying lizards and even a few dragons right and left, winning ninety-six percent of accounts receivable by her policy of dogged stubbornness mixed with patience. The very next day after I took her down to the facility, I entered a forest of paperwork that, while thinning after the first dense groves, wouldn't end until after her death.

I started out at the Division of Family Support. I'm sure I didn't actually make hundreds of drives to that building, but it certainly seemed it before the final decision on her case. I checked in and, after waiting my turn, was referred back to one of their caseworkers.

That marvelously thorough POA was handed over, skimmed, and accepted without question. The woman was sympathetic to my story as she pulled up her forms and started taking data, but within the first few questions, I jolted her badly when she asked the amount of Mom's Social Security. I replied that Mom had never filed for it. Never filed for it? Why on earth had she never filed for it? Because she thought the program was managed unethically and thus was morally against it.

The very idea that anyone eligible for Social Security had voluntarily turned her back on it was obviously incomprehensible to DFS. In that job, they were used to seeing hands always out, not hands clasped in refusal. The hardest part of that first interview was convincing the woman that, yes, Mom truly had *no* income, having deliberately avoided filing for what she easily could have had. Whatever there was had been donations from family. I had provided the trailer rent free, and we kids did help out financially as we could for food and such, but I had managed those funds myself, since Mom's financial ability had plummeted.

That became a far larger point than I had expected, that Mom herself did not hold and spend the money we gave her. Whose hands were on the funds apparently mattered a whole lot to DFS. I left that appointment with a list of things to bring back to the office, and prominently featured on it were statements from the family that funds provided in recent years had gone to me on Mom's behalf, not straight to her.

The biggest issue the DFS had, of course, was the Social Security. They wanted documentation that Mom truly was not receiving it. They also wanted her to start claiming hers monthly, thus whittling a little off the nursing home total they were being asked to cover. They wanted her to apply for disability, too. Mom would have thrown a fit before setting a foot inside a Social Security office, but I figured that battle was unwinnable. Her scruples would have to bow to the necessity of her care, though I had no intention of telling her what I was doing. So next, I proceeded to the Social Security office.

That first trip there was unforgettable. I've even had nightmares about it a few times. I took a number, explained the situation to the front triage desk when I was called, and received one of the rudest awakenings of Mom's whole illness, definitely the rudest paper-work-related one. I had brought the POA and the neuropsych assessment, but when I handed over the POA up front, the receptionist shook her head and said, "We don't accept POAs."

My expression probably mirrored that of the lady at DFS when I had told her Mom wasn't drawing Social Security. "You don't accept POAs? Everybody else has, including DFS."

She gave a governmental shrug. "Social Security does not accept POAs." She pulled out a form whatever from her slots. "This is our form. Your mother will need to sign this designating you as her representative. Until we have that, we cannot even discuss her case with you."

Ooo boy. I knew that my chances of getting Mom to sign anything prominently labeled Social Security Administration weren't good. Was this one form that I hadn't even known about going to topple the entire claim for assistance with the nursing home? I couldn't return to DFS and proceed there without documentation from Social Security and initiation of Mom's benefits.

While my mind galloped off into worst-case scenarios, Mom herself, speaking from memory, provided her old medical office advice. "Remember, Deb, bureaucracy respects persistence, even if they keep saying no or making excuses. You are wearing them down."

I was definitely holding up the line at the moment, something that always has bothered me. You should try to avoid inconveniencing innocent bystanders while fighting a battle. I asked to speak to one of the farther-backs, as I had seen some other people doing with complicated matters, and the receptionist, glad enough to pass this buck, gave me a new number and sent me to a new waiting area.

Three hours. It took three hours that afternoon, hours in which they kept saying they needed to speak to Mom or at least have her signature before they could even talk to me. I simply kept pointing to the cognitive testing with scores in the 0.02nd percentile and pleading that with things much worse now than back in the spring at that testing, she could no longer sign for anything. She was already in a nursing home, and this was urgent. I must admit, the thought occurred to me a few times that if I had gone to get Mom and returned with her, they would have gotten over wanting to talk to her in a hurry and gladly would have accepted me as a substitute. Mom in her right mind had hated Social Security. In her current state, I could only imagine the rant she would have delivered there.

Of course, retrieving Mom was out of the question. I fell back on stubbornness, a quality that is in ample supply in our family, though my version of it carried less fiery accompaniment than Mom's. I tried to remember that the people I was talking to were people as well as a governmental entity, and I was polite but relentless. I kept coming back to the reason of why we had to have this now, and I continued referencing the cognitive tests. She wasn't competent to sign anything by this point, as she was even worse than those figures now, and they were bad enough from months ago. Even if she did sign their form, her signature wouldn't mean anything legally. I was her daughter and only had her best interests at heart. Here was the official documentation of her mental capabilities, based on a complete competency screening, hours of testing by an independent expert. We had to get this started to apply for nursing home funding.

Finally, after what seemed like being locked in this red-tape stalemate forever, came three blessed words: "I believe you." At last, the person in front of me proved that she was, in fact, a person even if she did work at a governmental agency. She agreed to discuss Mom's case with me and try to help get the assorted balls rolling.

Now we could get down to actual figures. Starting the regular Social Security benefits was a cinch after that; Mom's complete work history was well known to their computer, and the paperwork took no time at all. It even could go directly to the nursing home toward her account there. The application for disability would be a much longer process, but the woman did copy the full neuropsych report, and we got the necessary paperwork started. She said she would request a rush on the decision, though Disability didn't always oblige. I also offered the POA for her to copy, and she shook her head, giving me a smile that was nearly as tired as my own after this ordeal. "I told you, Social Security does not accept POAs."

In the end, at least, they agreed to talk to me and start benefits and the disability application. That for that day was enough. I left the office with the statements DFS had wanted, the hard-fought prize for a full afternoon of bureaucracy. Mental note to self: if you ever plan to become demented, please be sure to fill out the Social Security form in advance specifying the date on which you intend to become demented and the person who will take over from you then.

Back to DFS. I presented signed statements from the family that we had given Mom *gifts*, not actual income, and that I had managed those. The Social Security paperwork was also handed over, though the disability claim was pending.

Here we met DFS's second detour sign on this road to nursing home funding. Their first had been to go to Social Security, go directly to Social Security, and do not collect any funds until after that. Now that I had gone to Social Security, they noticed something that hadn't been remarked upon in that first appointment. "She's only sixty-four."

Yes, she was. I knew she was young to have such extreme issues. I pointed out that the first problems I had noticed had started appearing when she was fifty-five and that she still had been sixty-three at the time of her abysmal performance on those cognitive tests in the spring.

Apparently, sixty-five is the magical age from the official point of view if you wish to enter a nursing home and seek assistance with the bills. Older than that, you're old enough to be in the short line. Younger, you have to get in the long line, and proving that you really need the placement is harder.

The cognitive testing was on our side, but then they asked for all other medical documentation through her decline. Trouble was, there wasn't any. Mom had been independent medically even in her prime, and in her illness, she had been downright paranoid. The appointment the day before her placement was her first with that doctor, and all that visit involved was the impending placement. That doctor took me at my word, backed up by the neuropsych report and the family emails, but she had barely performed any medical exam.

Mom's internist had been seen about every three to four years on average for a few decades, but that had slowed to a stop in the last several years. Even when she saw him, she wasn't the most compliant patient around. Her hypertension was a typical example of how Mom handled her own medical care. When the doctor had commented back in the 1990s that her blood pressure was getting high, she at first denied it. She was rushed, having a busy day, stressed with her parents, and it was an aberration. When he finally convinced her to keep a regular log, she discovered it was in fact high routinely, but then, after starting prescription meds, she began to worry about possible side effects. Then she started inventing side effects in what I think in retrospect was an early manifestation of her dementia. Then she flat out stopped taking the prescription and "cured" herself with herbs and vitamins. Then she stopped going for follow-up to avoid "hearing his arguments." She also, of course, stopped testing her own blood pressure once she started vitamins; since she knew she was going to be cured, there was no need to bother with continued testing. Just a waste of time.

I do think there can be value in natural medicine, though not completely replacing doctors, but refusing to keep testing her blood pressure, avoiding that mere two minutes in a store as she passed by the machine, was carrying things too far. Still, it was characteristic, even before the dementia. Mom always did have a tendency to carry things too far at times.

As I looked back from 2008, the last time she had actually had regular follow-up with a doctor on any sort of routine schedule and had followed instructions without a fight had been when she was pregnant with Daniel in 1983 and early 1984.

The end result was that there were very few medical records, and there were none for the years when DFS (and Disability, too, as it turned out) most wanted them. There was simply a long gap and then that cognitive screening in March 2008.

Down at the nursing home, they were trying to get medical data. Mom had an exam from the house doctor soon after her arrival, and they ordered a full array of lab work, including factors that can impact dementia. All of that came back perfectly normal. The only detail that stood out medically was her hypertension, not so cured after all, even though she was still on her vitamins, which had gone to the nursing home with her.

The quest for and provision of barely extant medical records occupied a few months during the claim. DFS and Disability both wanted much more than they got, the difference being that Disability at least sent me a list all at once of what they wished they had, while DFS specialized in dribbling out "just one more thing." Each time I returned to the office, they had come up with something else. Meanwhile, the bills from the nursing home rapidly rose into five figures. The nursing home never said a word, simply sent them to me, and as soon as her regular Social Security started, that contribution was paid directly to them monthly. It wasn't nearly enough, but it was something.

In the end, Disability denied the claim. I could have appealed it, but I had held out more hope for DFS all along. They had refused really to get rolling until Disability was determined, and a denial was at least an answer. I went back yet again to DFS and handed over the denial letter, and our speed of progress in the long line for Medicaid accelerated from a crawl to a stroll.

Finally, the decision came down. With the exception of the amount of her Social Security minus $35, the rest of the nursing home bill was covered by Medicaid. That $35 was Mom's personal allowance. The day I received that award letter was one of the few days I have actually broken down in tears (ones of gratitude that time) while opening the mail.

The forest of paperwork thinned a little at that point, but the path through it continued. For one thing, there was that $35 a month. That doesn't sound like much, but with a person who is institutionalized, never goes anywhere, and who has all room and board provided for, it can start adding up. It was the nursing home that warned me the first time her resident's fund hit a few hundred. Let that personal allowance build up far enough, and the limit is frighteningly low, and Medicaid would decide that Mom "had money." This would threaten her big award on the nursing home bills.

So I spent several years looking for ways to spend Mom's money for her. She got her beloved chocolate bars at first, extra large, an ample supply, but within the first year or two, she lost her desire for them. (Mom definitely was losing it more and more mentally.) Later, I ordered her a few nice sweaters from L. L. Bean when she started being cold all the time. These along with the one I had crocheted for her as a Christmas present years earlier gave her color choices. Mostly, I bought her cat things: cat shirts, cat pajamas, stuffed cats. One of the biggest hits of her whole illness was the cat quilt. That cost $170 and was well worth every penny for the smile it put on her face at a point when few things in the environment did anymore. With inventive shopping, I managed to keep that resident's fund under the limit throughout her stay.

Then there was the annual review form from the state. I grew to hate that. Multiple pages and one-size-fits-all, it contained such questions as listing all of your minor children at home and all of their fathers, sadly assuming that these were multiple. Then came the financial page: Do you have A? Do you have B? Do you have C? Clear on for a few dozen choices. Most of those Mom had never had in her life, much less now, but you had to fill out every last square. Nothing on the entire form could be left blank.

Every year, once it was turned in, a letter would come in reply after a few weeks. This letter would report that a decision had been reached on her claim, that we would be notified of the decision by separate cover in a few days, and that if I wished to appeal this decision (the one not specified yet), here was the appeal form to do it. Every year, upon reading that, I would shake my head and say, "Why?" What was the point of putting that information in two separate letters instead of in one? Did they just enjoy paying postage twice? Using twice as much paper? They easily could have said on the first letter, "We have reached a decision, and that decision is more/less/same." There was plenty of paper room left for another sentence. Also, how could I know if I wanted to appeal when I didn't even know yet from this first letter what I'd be appealing?

The decisions themselves were just as puzzling. Of course, if Social Security went up, her award would go down proportionally; that I understood. But other changes weren't as obvious. Once, for instance, the award was decreased two cents per month. Yes, two cents, twenty-four cents per year. It cost them more than those cents saved for the paperwork and people labor to get the adjustment made in the system. James' theory on that change was that higher-up bureaucrats now could beat their chests and announce that the amount spent on that budget line had been decreased, ergo the state was saving money and being more financially responsible.

It was alternately exasperating, frustrating, and amusing, but beyond all of that, I was still grateful. Almost all her bills during the nursing home years were covered, and the amounts on some of those non-bills I would receive were staggering. The need was met. Mom would have hated knowing how, but she had been a working, productive member of society all her life as long as she could. We never asked for aid until we had no other choice; when we needed it, it was there. I appreciated it.

Mom never knew how the nursing home was paid for. She did ask me a few times over the years, always phrased as a worry that the bills were being a burden on us, her children. I didn't mention Social Security or Medicaid; I just told her that it was taken care of and that we were not having to do it ourselves. That always reassured her. In her prime, she would have pushed on to ask where the buck did stop, but in her dementia, on this topic at least, she would accept my reassurance. She was most concerned financially about being a burden to us.

Some days, she would pull open her nightstand drawer and take out some quarters. "I won this at bingo," she would say as she pushed the coins into my hand. "You take it. It will help a little bit for the bills." I would take the quarters and solemnly thank her, and she would smile her familiar sweet smile with the "accomplishment" edge of satisfaction in it. For as long as she was capable of joining the bingo games, she gave me her winnings, always designated as a payment toward her care or my expenses in coming to visit her.

The quarters I didn't forward to the nursing home. On those days, I would stop at a convenience store on the way home and put her quarters toward what, before she forgot it, had been her lifelong favorite. Then I would sit out in the car with the memories for company and raise a Special Dark bar to the most thoughtful, determined, feisty, remarkable woman I have ever known.

# 11.

## *Settling and Sorting*

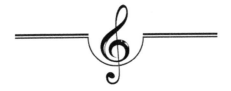

M om's peaceful and compliant transition to the nursing home didn't last too long. I went down the very next day after her placement to visit, the first of literally hundreds of such trips, and she seemed a little more restless but still oriented to and accepting the change. Within the next day or so, however, she escaped, not wandering but apparently deliberately leaving, as she admitted when found. Mom had never once tried to leave Erdenheim either intentionally or in confusion, but she wasted no time in taking off from the facility. The nursing home, with their multigenerational acquaintance with our family, well remembered Granddaddy. He had given them fits before the locked unit was built, often requiring the police to track him down. The home decided that the apple might not fall far from the tree, and they jumped Mom immediately all the way up to the highest level, moving her to the locked unit and tagging her with a WanderGuard for good measure. Her stay in her first room had lasted only three days.

I had planned to visit to have lunch with her every week, something she herself had done with her parents for years, and I hoped that the familiarity of that routine would reach her. Daniel went with me to those weekly visits initially, and that first Friday when we arrived for lunch, she was already up on the locked unit. She was even more restless then and had started the routine of "pacing" the hall in her wheelchair, which she kept up intermittently until a few weeks before her death.

Then on Sunday night, not yet a week from placement, came the first extra phone call from staff. Mom was insisting on talking to me, the aide said, and they couldn't settle her down. When they put Mom on the line, she sounded completely bewildered. She had been waiting for me, she said, but I hadn't come yet, and when was I going to pick her up so we could go home? I explained that she lived there now, and her reply was poignantly puzzled. "Do they know that?" All memory of the previous week, of the doctor and our conversations, had left the building. Like Rip van Winkle, she had just woken up in a new world.

I did my best to reassure her. She was in a good place, and yes, they knew she was there. I would be back regularly to visit. She didn't argue that night (though we were to have some intense debates through the years on the subject of leaving). She was simply confused. After she seemed to have settled down, though still disoriented, I asked to speak to the aide again and suggested playing some of her classical music.

This became the pattern over the next several months. Mom had times when the situation was brand new. Then there were other times when she knew where she was and didn't want to stay. On the third hand, she might be fairly peaceful.

The nursing home was enjoyable in several ways for her. While we both loved Erdenheim, it is remote, to put it mildly, and there is next to no socialization. If you want society, you have to drive a bit. Once she became unable to leave the farm, she was very isolated, even with two of her kids living right there. Confined largely to the house by her legs, she spent basically all day at the computer, which she still could use. Mom had loved news all her life, dating back to the newspapers from which Granddaddy taught her to read, but reading news stories and alleged news stories on the Internet for twelve hours a day is not ideal for a person with dementia. I think that the isolation mixed with the politics and not-always-accurate news feeds helped shape some of her paranoia and delusions.

At the facility, there were people with whom she could interact. The events planner provided a wealth of activities, music, and remember-when games. Even on the locked unit with the worst cases, they tried to give them gentle, positive things to do, and they let her off the locked unit for a few hours on good days to attend some of the activities in the general population. All that was very good for her.

Then there was the library. The nursing home had a large library, several thousand volumes; in fact, we had borrowed that room for years to have the family birthday parties, Thanksgiving, and Christmas during Grandmother and Granddaddy's stay. Ten people could have eaten Thanksgiving dinner in there comfortably at the large table without taking up more than a fourth of the room. Mom had been too busy with logistics on those former days to have time to enjoy the books, but now, she took to that library like a duck to water. At home, she had loved reading science and psychology for self-improvement and science fiction and fantasy for pleasure. This library, though, was very heavily tilted to soft, gentle romantic fiction. No difficulties existed that could not be solved in a few hundred pages, and they unfailingly lived happily ever after. These books were soothing, no doubt intentionally for that population, and Mom, who once would have thought them not challenging enough, now appreciated them.

The book cart from the library came through the locked unit weekly and usually left her five or six, and she would read them fully, too. Her reading speed still was barely compromised; she could easily in her initial years there put away five 300-page books in a week. Staff took to marking "pw" in pencil inside the flaps to indicate which she had read so as not to duplicate in picking out next week's selection for her. To this day, I'm sure the majority of the books down in that library bear Mom's mark.

Mom also discovered TV. She had never had time for much TV, and, in fact, there were many years growing up when we didn't even have one in the house. Now, though, they had movie nights at the facility, and all patients had a private TV in their rooms. She especially enjoyed getting acquainted with Judge Judy.

Her legs started improving tremendously, and she even walked a good bit with her walker (or without it, to the staff's chagrin), though she still used the wheelchair for long distances. Throughout the rest of her life, her walking would wax and wane, seemingly more tied to her mental health than to her physical.

Still, the restlessness was there at times and slowly increased. She began actively lashing out on occasion. At the first care plan meeting with the staff, two months after her placement, they gave me her long-handled back scratcher, her grabber thing with suction cups, and her cane. These had had to be confiscated; she used them to poke or whack at others when she grew impatient and agitated.

She still made a few attempts at escape. It was impossible now due to the secure environment, but she tried nonetheless. She also wrote a letter to Daniel that I found on her nightstand one day when I was visiting alone. That email I had found to the family on her computer, the one she was working on the night after that doctor's appointment and the night before her placement, had looked like a draft, and I wasn't sure it had ever been sent. I knew this letter at the nursing home hadn't been sent. The address written on the back of it (no envelope, simply the paper folded into thirds) was Daniel, Erdenheim, Missouri, correctly written out on three lines, and the return address was Mom, Manor, Missouri.

In that letter, she was oriented to her location and even described it remarkably accurately, including highway numbers to get there. She said that I had put her there to get rid of her, and she was asking Daniel to drive down and pick her up. Since I didn't want her to live with me anymore, they could find another place. "We can work something out," is the line I particularly remember. She provided directions, although he, of course, had been down there many times to the family events with the grandparents and also had visited her by then. I read that letter over, and then I simply threw it away. It was written by the disease, not by her. As much as the misunderstandings hurt, I never lost sight of that fact.

Music could still calm her down, but she got frustrated with her little tape/CD player as she forgot how to use it, and she "disciplined" it for not working, eventually going too far. Several times during the rest of her life, those players had to be replaced. A sad smile would accompany my head shake of frustration each time I bought another one, because in a way, even if carried too far now, that action was *so* Mom. She had had little patience with electronics all her life, and many times, I had seen her spank a computer. She never had trouble figuring out new programs, but the general computer moodiness that most of the world accepts with a wry shrug she took as a challenge. She really did believe that we had God-given dominion over our own inventions as well as over the world.

Meanwhile back at the farm, the careful sorting out of a lifetime's possessions started. The hardest thing for me was going through her purse. I had looked in her purse for something many times over the years at her own request. This time, however, was infinitely different. Little things, routine things, painfully familiar things pricked my heart, such as the leather P that she always had on her keys for so many years that was starting to split around the edges. I held that P and wished for some key to unlock this situation and remove the obstacle. None appeared, but I still treasured the memories. I carefully tucked the P away in a drawer for myself.

I sent a "speak now or hold your peace" email to the family saying that I was starting to sort Mom's worldly goods, and if anybody had ever wanted anything, this was their opportunity. Almost everyone did want something. James and Beth wanted the quilts made by Mom's grandmother. Daniel wanted the rocking chair. Michael chose Granddaddy's desk, a solid structure with as much character and integrity as the man himself had displayed throughout his life. Vicki had always wanted a tall oak bookcase built by Mom's grandfather, who had been a carpenter. Rena had her eye on the cast iron skillets. For myself, I took the cedar chest, which had been a wedding present to Mom from her parents. I also took the Flying painting, and many times over the years, I would stand and look at that dark-haired girl at the full extent of her swing, head back, so alive and passionate.

Much of the routine furniture simply stayed in the trailer, as Daniel took it over and continued living there, though he did pay me rent from the point of Mom's placement in the nursing home. He adopted Mom's final two cats, Tablet and Grace, and often, we reassured her as to their well-being.

What took the most time to sort out were the pictures. All her life Mom had had a filing system, if you could call it that, of tossing things into a box mentally labeled, "To be put into photo albums whenever I get around to it." She never did. Meanwhile, as boxes became full or were misplaced, other boxes were started. Often more than one was being filled at the same time. There was no system or date arrangement; pictures from the 1960s could be side by side with ones decades later. Going through all of it took me well over a year.

There was also no labeling. With the fresh example of Mom's dementia in mind, I set about remedying that as soon as I could, before someone else died or became incapable and we lost that knowledge bank forever. I started scanning the best pictures—not everything, because eight of the same cat in nearly the same pose or three of the same tree just planted were a case of over-kill. But I picked out the ones of the people, especially, and began to scan them, building a disc. When it was full I sent it to the whole family, resulting in multiple copies in widely scattered places. Some of the photos were damaged from the house fire; I'm sure others had been fully destroyed in the fire, because there were gaps in subject matter. There are very few, for instance, of me as a young child. Full storage boxes at the time of the fire had been elsewhere, but the current box from that era was quite damaged. When my picture scanning project was finished, with the multiple copies distributed around America, nothing short of a nuclear doomsday would wipe those images out of existence.

I also set about identifying the subjects, emailing everybody with the mysteries. Vicki was the greatest ally there, having known several of the people in the older pictures. What she couldn't come up with, she forwarded to the Arkansas relatives. We were probably able to identify ninety-eight percent of the people in the pictures, but there remained a few question marks at the end, someone's life, one who had mattered to our circle, now completely unknown. Please, please, label your pictures as you take them.

There were also moments of nostalgia and of humor in that project. I sometimes, as I found a shot I particularly liked, would email a scan to the family not as a mystery but simply as a memory to be appreciated together. One day, I came across a shot obviously taken on Easter Sunday, judging from the clothes. Grandmother, Granddaddy, Mom, and Vicki were standing in front of their car, with only part of the car visible peeking out behind the family. Vicki looked about six, Mom about sixteen. Neat shot. I emailed it to everyone to enjoy.

I received three replies, and the third one cracked me up. Rena responded with, "Nice family picture!" Vicki said, "We all look so young." Dad replied, not even mentioning the people, with "That's a," and he named the exact model and year of the car, exclamation point included.

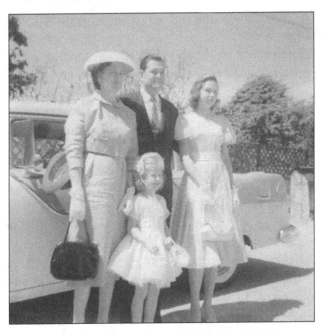

**The family in their Easter best – and cameo appearance by their car.**

There were a few other items in the picture boxes, too, little notes or bits of paperwork. One of those especially touched me. When I was young, we kids would wait with excitement for the Sears Wish Book each Christmas, and we would go through and dream shop. We knew that not everything we wanted would be received, but it was fun to imagine. I found, in Mom's handwriting, a list obviously made from some year's Wish Book. This was her own dream shopping list, with a column for each of her three children (this note far predated Daniel). The presents that she wanted to give us surpassed by a large margin what we had wanted for ourselves. A mother's dream, written down in hopeful love, then folded and put aside as she returned to the realities of life.

Then there were the Piano Rules. This long piece of poster board held Mom's handwritten and carefully enumerated list of how children should approach her beloved instrument with due deference. At the bottom, it concluded, "Violators will be prosecuted, spanked, fined, harassed, and will otherwise incur the wrath of the management." I could hear the words in her voice. Years later, that list went to her funeral and was displayed up front along with the pictures. Several people there asked for copies. I ultimately had it framed and hung proudly above my own piano.

Upon finishing the picture sorting, I selected several that gave a chronicle of Mom's life. Baby pictures. Mom growing up. With her children. With her cats. With her piano. The picture from that Fish Feathers recital, though it was taken far after that point, when she was absorbed with full determination in the music. Mom with the sweater I crocheted for her in 1989.

Growing older. At Erdenheim, the shadow of the illness now beginning to fall across her face. The last picture chosen was Mom reading the Christmas story from the Bible at Christmas 2007, her last one at home. I had those made into a tribute video, seeking professional help editing it, and set them to me singing "No More Night," her favorite song about heaven. That was intended for—and, years later, used at—her funeral. She had asked me once to sing "No More Night" then, and I didn't think I could get through it. But the video would be a good substitute, and I thought she would have liked it.

Words at the beginning and end of the video bookended the pictures. The opening screen said, "Paulette Webb. Mother, Sister, Best Friend." Then it quoted Philippians 1:3: "I thank my God in all my remembrance of you." At the end, after that final shot of Mom reading the Christmas story, it said, "Looking forward to singing with you again in heaven's choir."

I didn't show it to her. She was too restless at that point for the reminder of the world outside and the life she no longer enjoyed, and later, she was too confused to appreciate it. The video was finished and put aside, waiting, as her life now seemed to be waiting. Many dark and some bright days remained ahead before it was to be used.

That first Thanksgiving, two months after her placement, we had portable Thanksgiving dinner (turkey sandwiches and chips) down in the library. I wanted to try to keep the tradition going that we always maintained throughout Grandmother and Granddaddy's stay of having local family celebrations there so Mom could be included. The gatherings dwindled after a couple of attempts; seeing Mom was simply too painful of an ongoing change for the relatives, I think. But that first Thanksgiving, Vicki came and Daniel. In separate cars from our separate schedules, we convened.

I arrived early to collect Mom. The library was a very long wheelchair ride from the unit, a few buildings over in the basement, including a steep ramp connecting those buildings. She hadn't been to the library herself since her arrival, as it was such a trek. I wheeled her over, and she roll-ambled around the shelves, looking at the books. She was in a good mood that day, fairly settled, reasonably oriented to place and to Thanksgiving. We sang some and also joked while waiting for Vicki; Vicki had been notoriously late all her life and was almost always the last one to arrive at a family event.

Finally, Vicki came, bringing with her the sandwich tray and drinks; I had brought chips. She descended the stairs from the parking lot into the basement. She hadn't seen Mom since her daughter Jennifer's wedding in 2006. There were my constant updates, of course, but no words could fully convey the decline. Even on a good day, looking at Mom now was heartbreaking.

Vicki showed not a ruffle right then, greeted Mom with a smile and a hug, and then put down her first load, saying there were other things in the car. I ducked out of the library myself to help collect them. As I came back down the stairs with hands full, I met Vicki going up, and she stopped dead halfway. We faced each other there on the staircase, frozen in midjourney. "My God," she said. It was not a curse but a prayer. I nodded. "It's bad," I replied. Vicki reached out and put a hand on my shoulder, a silent acknowledgment that the words were inadequate.

After a brief moment, we split apart, and I continued back down to the library. Vicki reappeared with the last of the sacks a minute later, and we sorted out the meal and sat down. Mom was pleasant, chatty. It could have been any routine family meeting over the years—but it wasn't and never would be again.

Then we joined hands and bowed our heads and gave thanks.

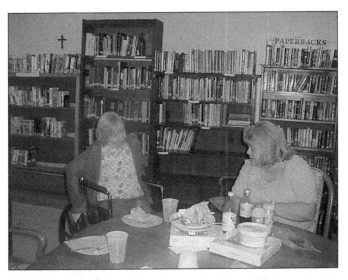

**Mom and Vicki, Thanksgiving 2008.**

# 12.

## *Transfer*

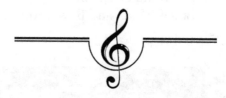

Getting a call from the nursing home in the middle of the week was rarely good news. The call in late March was no exception.

"We have a problem," said the Director of Nursing, getting straight to the point. "We can't keep your mother here anymore."

My heart plummeted to my toes. "Why?"

"The outbursts are getting worse. Yelling, throwing things, even violence. It's more frequent."

I had no response at first. I knew that on bad days, Mom was horribly difficult to manage. Even in her prime of life, she could be volatile at times when frustrated, though she had never been violent toward people. In previous years, she had directed her annoyance toward uncooperative objects, slain a few lizards, or simply attacked a hard physical project to work off steam. How much more frustrated must she be now? She knew, at least on many days, that something was badly wrong. I could see it in her eyes, hear it in her voice, even though she never could quite manage the step of assigning the cause to illness on her own part. Instead, she lashed out. She had broken electronics by this point, and the cane, back scratcher, and reacher had long since been confiscated. I had dreaded her turning with more vigor on other people, but I'd been afraid this might be coming.

The Director of Nursing continued. She wanted Mom transferred to the inpatient psychiatric hospital up in the city. If they could get her stabilized, she could come back to the Manor later, but she would have to be more manageable than she was currently. Then, with the compassion mixed with knowledge of details that was so characteristic of that facility, the DON went on to bring up a point I had not even considered. "Her birthday is coming up very soon."

"April 9," I confirmed.

"That is going to make a big difference. She becomes eligible for Medicare then. So what I'd like to do is to try to keep her here a few more days. If we can wait until the ninth for transfer, the paperwork and finances for the hospital will be so much easier for you." She paused, then moved on steadily, deftly walking the tightrope between care for one patient and responsibility to the rest. Her suggestion was to sedate Mom for those few days, buying us the necessary time.

To date, I had bent over backwards trying to honor Mom's frequently and vehemently stated wishes throughout her life to avoid prescription medication. Everything so far, the power company episode, the delusions, the horrible summer of 2008, her increasing restlessness and frustration at the nursing home, had been on no prescribed meds at all. But I knew that era of her life was over. Safety, that of others and of herself, now trumped her wishes. The disease had forced our hand.

I agreed and authorized this plan. There was no other option. She certainly couldn't come back home to Erdenheim. I had hit the limits of capability back in 2008, and if Mom had been beyond me then, she certainly still was. She couldn't stay at the nursing home in her current state. I did tell the DON how much I appreciated the facility letting us buy time until Medicare kicked in and for not insisting on a transfer right away.

So Mom went onto regular doses of Ativan, deliberately trying for this short term to slow her down. The effect was obvious on my next visit. They were having to lie to her about the meds; everything was presented to her as "vitamins." On days when she refused to accept even "vitamins," they gave her laced pudding or applesauce. The drug did put a chemical brake on her as we needed, and they tried to keep it at the minimum effective level.

I had had other plans for Mom's birthday for a while: I wanted to take her a cat. Her own two cats were doing well with Daniel, but unfortunately, neither was a great candidate for being stuffed in a carrier, hauled an hour and a half, and then brought out in a strange environment full of clinical smells and sounds and even disoriented people.

Calling the roll of my own cats, which Mom also knew already, of course, from living on Erdenheim, I had concluded that the best candidate was Tenuto. Tenuto was a seal-point Siamese, purebred. I've always loved the breed and had had several Siamese mixes in childhood. Tenuto was my third full Siamese, and contrary to all stereotypes, she was nearly unflappable, possessing a lot of "whateveritude." Her housemate Rosalind, on the other hand, my second pure Siamese, was an extreme diva with zero tolerance for anything or anybody out of the routine and would have turned into a fur tornado in nothing flat at the facility. Over the years, through several cats, I've concluded that Siamese, like people and like other cats, have different personalities among themselves. There are quiet ones, even if those are the minority; my first full Siamese was one of the quietest cats I've ever known. There are calmer ones (Tenuto) and more dramatic ones (Rosalind). The main thing about Siamese in my experience is that whatever root personality they have, it is dialed up to maximum. They are much more intense than non-Siamese in their individually varying ways.

So the lot fell to Tenuto, and I was practicing her with a collar and leash. The nursing home had approved a feline but wanted her under control. The cat thought this was odd but did not object.

On Mom's sixty-fifth birthday, Tenuto and I headed down to the nursing home. Mom was pathetic that day and looked worse than before, though the dose on the Ativan hadn't been increased. She was slumped over in her chair, staring at her lap. You couldn't even see her face when standing in front of her as her hair fell over it. I carefully placed the cat in her arms in the wheelchair, and her hands grasped her, then automatically started petting. Mom's head came up a little. Tenuto, who for all her level-headedness usually did have a limit to laps, preferring a short stay and then an exit on her own timing, sat there perfectly content and started to purr.

One of the nurses tapped me and asked for a few words privately. I considered the situation, then tied the leash to the arm of the wheelchair. Tenuto never objected. Keeping a wary eye out, I retreated a short way.

They had the transfer papers and wanted me to sign them. Right then and there, I did, signing papers committing Mom to a psychiatric hospital on the actual day of her sixty-fifth birthday. April 9, 2009, is another date that, like February 22, 2008, I don't think I'll ever forget in this life unless I myself develop dementia.

The paperwork done, the nurse said they would set the wheels into motion and get her moved as soon as possible. I could expect a call from the intake evaluator from the psych hospital, probably even that day.

Back to Mom and Tenuto, who was still a purring Siamese statue. I wished Mom a happy birthday, sang to her, and then after a while reloaded the cat and left. There was nothing more I could do. There was nothing more they could do. Everything, everybody, has limits. That, back in September, had been one of the bitterest lessons for me. The taste wasn't any better now.

Once back in Kipling with the doors closed, I opened the Pet Taxi to reach in and scratch Tenuto's ears and thank her for being such a star. She promptly moved out into my lap, and this cat who preferred her lap time in short doses sat there the entire hour and a half drive home, purring and looking at me with such solicitude that it brought tears to my eyes. She knew. With as much understanding as a feline could possess, she knew that Mom was sick, and she knew that I was heartbroken, and she tried her best to comfort me. Thank you, Lord, for the gift of animals.

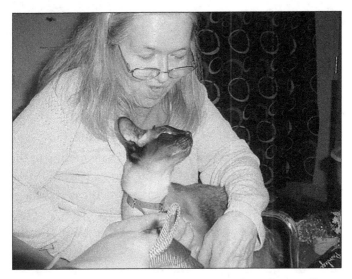

**Tenuto visited Mom many times over the years and was always wonderful with her.**

The intake evaluator from the hospital called me later that same day. He had been down to see Mom and had read the chart, and he wanted a full history, my version. I gave him the whole story, the slowly advancing memory decline and then the days since February 2008 when memory decline was no longer the primary problem. He commented how young she was for such extreme issues. Of course, she was drugged up that day and not really able to be personally interviewed and tested, but he did confirm later on in her hospitalization that she was the most advanced case for her age that he had ever seen.

I went down to visit as soon as I could the day after that. Mom was at the hospital, definitely not drugged up now, and was unsettled. She wasn't explosive, not that day, but she wasn't happy. Her first comment when

I entered was, "You found me." I promised her that we knew where she was and that I would be there as often as I could.

Then came more paperwork, of course, signing forms for the hospital and talking to the staff in person. They wanted to do a thorough workup medically as well as psychiatrically, because they suspected given her age that something else might be contributing to the dementia. I was all for that, and in the next week Mom underwent the most comprehensive medical testing of her life: CAT scan of the brain, all sorts of blood tests, ruling out toxins and deficiencies, ruling out a few diseases other than dementia that could impact mental function and reality perception.

In the end, they found nothing, and they were trying hard to find something. All the results from multiple texts came back negative. The official diagnosis they landed back on was Alzheimer's disease, early presentation, with hallucinations and delusions.

With nothing but that left to treat, we had to accept the inevitable. Mom went onto antipsychotics as well as meds that sometimes slow memory loss. For the rest of her life, from that hospitalization on, she would be on several prescriptions. Getting her stabilized at the right levels took some serious effort (and would prove to be a continuing roller coaster throughout the remainder of her life), but she did start becoming easier to manage without being simply overly sedated as she had seemed on her birthday while we were buying time for Medicare to kick in.

For a few months, back before the question of the transfer ever came up, we had been trying to arrange for the whole family to visit her on her birthday. This proved impossible on the day itself due to schedules of the two nonlocal brothers, in particular Michael, who on the East Coast had the longest drive. The target date wound up being several days later. She was in the hospital at that point, but we kept to the plan and just changed the destination.

Earlier that evening, we met at a restaurant in the city and ate together. Many of these people, Vicki and Michael, for instance, hadn't seen each other in years, and the conversation was strictly catching up on the details of the various lives. The topic of Mom during dinner was almost completely avoided. Of course, everybody had had the weekly-at-minimum updates for months and much more frequent ones during the recent hospitalization. There wasn't any catching up to do regarding Mom.

Then we trekked in convoy over to the hospital. The psych hospital was a completely different world from the nursing home. There were limits on visitors at one time, and you had to call from the other side of the locked door to state your credentials and request entrance. We started dutifully going in two at a time, but when the staff found out that this was actually a birthday gathering, even if not on her birthday, they bent the rules and let us in en masse, simply requesting that we be quiet. Mom was glad to see everyone but a bit overwhelmed by the crowd, I think. Dad and Rena ducked out early after a few minutes to ease the number of people present and give the kids and their families time. We initially had planned on a birthday cake, but Rena had a marvelous idea when it became obvious that this gathering would be in the hospital, not at the nursing home. She suggested cupcakes instead, much more portable and easier to pass out. Mom enjoyed the visit, but there was an overlying fragility about her, such a painful change from her forceful but compassionate personality through her life.

Afterward, we left her. I do remember that Melanie, Michael's wife, told me quietly as we were leaving the building that she truly appreciated the updates and everything I'd been doing. Thank you, Melanie. I needed that that evening. As it says in Proverbs, "A word fitly spoken is like apples of gold in pictures of silver."[19]

With a few final goodbyes, we all got back into our respective cars. This couldn't be a long visit; it had required logistical gymnastics to get it coordinated at all. As it turned out, that evening would be the last time in Mom's life that the entire family would be assembled at the same time.

A few days after the birthday gathering, Mom was discharged, and the Manor agreed to take her back. The long list of prescriptions and orders went with her. With the exception of a couple of hours out for a few specialist doctor appointments, the nursing home would be her constant environment for the remaining seven years of her life.

# 13.

## *The Roller Coaster*

Mom never was fond of roller coasters. She greatly enjoyed driving along a winding, hilly road, even commenting on those that would make a good roller coaster with track simply installed alongside the pavement, but there was a huge difference between driving such a course herself and being strapped into a cart and propelled along one. The thing she hated about amusement park rides was the loss of control.

From her return to the nursing home in spring 2009 through the end of her life, she was on a roller coaster. She wasn't driving, and I'm sure she was scared by it far more than she would have been by any ride designer's most ambitious creation. All she, all any of us could do was hang on as it rocketed around curves, slowly climbed, teased with brief calms, then hurtled down to new depths.

The medicines definitely helped. The moods, the explosiveness, the agitation were blunted somewhat, and fortunately she never became outright violent again. Sometimes, she even seemed to be doing well. The most challenging reality about Mom's case, however, was its total inconsistency. The doses that had worked well for months could suddenly be wrong, requiring readjusting, then needing adjusting back later to the original level. There seemed to be no rhyme or reason to it.

Her speech skills remained excellent up until about the last year and a half of her life, and she was very good at conversation and interacting with people. Shortly after her return from the psych hospital stay, they even moved her back off the locked unit. She still was tagged with a WanderGuard, but she didn't try to escape, not for a few years, at least, and she was so much more advanced in speech and activity than most of the residents on the locked unit that they thought the general population might be less frustrating for her. This was yet another tightrope to be walked; she was ahead of almost all the other advanced dementia patients in speech, but she was far behind the general population in reality orientation and common sense. Her memory continued to decline slowly, but it continued to be the least of her problems now.

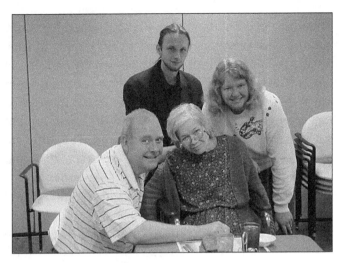

**Michael, Daniel, and me with Mom on her
sixty-sixth birthday.**

She did enjoy the general floor, and we agreed that
the move was good for her right then. She played bingo,
attended activities, and loved the music. They did have
some false starts at pairing her up with a roommate, but
after the initial failures, she wound up with one who,
to my surprise, suited her to a T. That woman was all
but unconscious, present only by breathing. She didn't
speak much, didn't interact much, and was a rag doll
positioned in either bed or chair, much as Grandmother
had been in her last months. There was no need to put
her on the locked ward, as she never did anything, much
less tried to escape. She simply existed. I would have
expected Mom to get bored or frustrated living with her,
but Mom could still surprise me. She was marvelous
with that lady.

She even learned—quickly and accurately—her
roommate's very subtle nonverbal cues and often

pushed the call button to alert the staff when her room-mate needed attention. The staff rapidly grew to trust her judgment on this. I was talking with one of the nurses one day and mentioned that it was odd that Mom enjoyed living with this woman so much more than with someone she could talk to, and the nurse replied that it was her conclusion that Mom needed a roommate far below her own level so that she could feel maternal and/or responsible for her. That was an excellent point, and the staff tried to stick with it as much as they could in the future after that woman ultimately moved on. Yes, Mom did well with socialization outside of her room and with responsibilities, even if self-assigned, within it. She had always possessed both strong maternal and responsibility streaks.

Her walking improved at first, never back to base-line and never totally steady, but better. They tried to let her walk every day as exercise but only with super-vision. Her stamina was still shot, and she used the wheelchair for longer distances, such as to the dining room, but she absolutely refused to let anybody push her except me. The staff often commented on that. Mom was fiercely self-propelled, and she would bite workers' heads off verbally if they tried to help, even up the ramp.

Ah, the ramp. That was a momentary bright glimmer in those dark days, a diamond. Mom's room was up a hall that had two distinct levels due to the lay of the ground on which it was built. Her room was on the upper end, and the nurses' station and T intersection with the main hall to the dining room were on the lower end. Between the levels was a ramp, not nearly as long or steep as the one between buildings that led to the library but still a definite slope.

Mom would pause at the top of it, push off, and then hold her hands and feet up while calling, "Whee!" as the wheelchair raced down the ramp. She then would drop her feet and stop herself right at the intersection at the base of it. Not once did she crash into the wall on the other side of the hall, though staff would cringe visibly as they watched her brief moment of ecstasy. Warnings were fruitless. "Paulette, be careful." "I *am* being careful. I know what I'm doing." "Don't crash and hurt yourself." "I have no intention of it." The whole thing was classic Mom. For that short distance and not-extreme slope, she could do it with control, and she reveled in it. Watching her, I often thought of the girl on the swing, head back, hair streaming, lost in the pure joy of motion, flying.

On the return from the dining hall, it was a different story. Then, the ramp was going up, of course, and no charge with abandon was possible. Instead, it was a long haul, one laborious wheel turn and paddle step at a time. She would be panting with the effort. But even then, she refused assistance except from me. I often pushed her back up that ramp, asking first if she'd like help, and she would accept without complaint and thank me for the offer. Let a staff member ask if she would like help, and she'd annihilate them. She could do things *herself*. If some poor good Samaritan took hold of the handles behind her anyway, she would detect the added strength at once and protest not only verbally but physically, dropping her feet farther and deliberately blocking the wheels.

But she did let me assist her. That, too, was a diamond. There were still occasional days and would continue to be when I was the diabolical daughter who had cast her off, but there were also many moments when we seemed to reach each other in spite of the illness, not with our old seamlessness but still with a modified sort of partnership. She also would calm down most for me on her days of worst agitation. The staff commented on that. They tried very hard to handle situations themselves, and calls from Mom were rare. However, on the worst days when all other efforts had failed, they would put her on the line to talk to me. When those calls came, it did usually help, and even if upset, she wasn't quite as much in turmoil by the end of our conversation.

On days of good weather, both mentally and meteorologically, I would take her outside for the first few years for a roll around the grounds, looking at trees and flowers, talking. I would ask which way she wanted to go, but she most often left it up to me, and sometimes she would attach an addendum to that statement. "I trust you." Those moments were balm to be stored up and applied on the other kind of days, the ones when she would accuse me of kicking her off Erdenheim just because I wanted it for myself or of siding with the world against her.

The subject of food became an increasing challenge in her nursing home years. Mom had been somewhat of a picky eater through life anyway; her menu card had printed at the top in capitalized and bolded type next to her name, "VERY SELECTIVE." In the nursing home, she took this to new heights. A few times, she basically went on a hunger strike, apparently seizing the one area in her life she could still control. Those were challenging periods, because we weren't ever going to force her or feed her by tubes or IVs. If she truly decided to starve herself, she did have that option. The

210

staff had the patience of saints working with her. Her weight, like her mind, traveled through some big hills and steep drops during those trying years, but then it would recover some of the lost ground.

She went through a long period where she decided that the only food she would eat was a pimento cheese sandwich. I took to calling these SASs: Sole Acceptable Sandwiches. The staff dutifully made her a SAS on days when she refused anything else, and she would usually eat at least part of that. I tried to leave church early at least once a month to arrive for the usual Sunday visit in time to eat with her and monitor the food situation. At first, she was quite chatty during meals, enjoying the conversation. Later, it became harder physically with difficulty finding her mouth, and intense concentration was needed. By the last months, I deliberately tried not to get there while she was eating, as any distraction at all cost her calories.

She also had a few food-related fixations that cropped up. One of those concerned grape jelly. She started stockpiling grape jelly from the dish in the middle of the table that contained butter, jelly, and spreads. Always grape, no other flavor. Eventually, she branched out and scavenged at other tables to acquire their grape jelly, too. She ate this straight, not spread on anything. In fact, one day when I suggested that she put it on her biscuit, she looked at me as if this was the most ludicrous statement she had ever heard and asked why on earth she would ever want to do that. She even carried grape jelly out, taking several packets back to her room because, "I might want a snack." Later on, it was bananas; she arrived early for breakfast specifically to cruise the entire room and take bananas from the fruit baskets at each table. She didn't eat all of the bananas, simply collected them. The staff would simply shrug and make sure there was extra grape jelly and plenty of bananas.

The delusions continued, never entirely under control even on antipsychotics. Regularly, she would come up with what I privately referred to as employee of the month, although it wasn't a positive title. Most of the candidates actually held the position longer than a month; she would switch three or four times a year. Employee X, who might or might not actually exist and work there, "had it in for" Mom for some reason and set out "to teach (her) a lesson." These stories were so far out of reason that they were obviously delusional. Also, many of these employees of the month did not match any description of anyone who had ever worked there past or present. Mom even admitted that nobody else ever saw those "because they're sneaky." As for the employees of the month who actually did exist, that same staff member might have been one of her favorites six months before and might be again six months after. There was no correlation with reality.

One of these was the beauty shop lady. This woman had worked there at the nursing home a few days a week for years and had even done Grandmother's hair, so Mom knew her already. Mom at first enjoyed getting her hair done. Then one day, they came to take her for her appointment, and she flipped out. Nope, that woman was diabolical, had it in for her, and even used "evil scissors." The staff relented, since obviously she wasn't going to be able to be worked on in the beauty shop that day, and for months, Mom didn't get her hair cut. During this time, it grew out, eventually longer than I had ever seen it in my life. I liked it. It was beautiful: long, flowing, silky, and softly silver. Even when the beauty shop lady passed on the title of employee of the month to someone else, and Mom had no memory at all that there had ever been an issue with getting her hair done, I asked them simply to trim it up but leave it long.

She wore it that way to the end of her life, and the staff enjoyed playing around with it. There were five or six different styles I saw in rotation, not applied at the beauty shop but arranged for the day by whichever aide dressed her. She might have it in French braids, or in a bun, or pulled to one side with a barrette. It really looked attractive, and I complimented them several times through the years on the special effort they clearly took for the patients' appearances. "People still ought to look nice," was the reply given. Even with Mom's near-comatose roommate, I cannot count the times I saw them, when they came to take her to the feeding room, first comb her hair and then put on her jewelry. That woman apparently had always worn jewelry; she had a lot of it. They made sure that she still wore jewelry, even if she was no longer aware of it, and she always looked as nice as she could when they took her out of the room.

The privacy curtain was another major delusion that took up months. Mom became convinced that it was killing her plants in the room. I don't mean by lack of light; Mom had claustrophobia, and the privacy curtain was almost never drawn. If it was pulled around, Mom would object immediately. She wanted it tucked way back behind her bed, and it was nowhere near coming between the plants and the window. The true problem with Mom's plants was that Mom herself was watering them to death, but any effort to explain that only led to agitation. No, it was the privacy curtain, which by simply being in the room cast a spell on them.

I finally managed to find a few plants that were advertised to be as tough as nails, nearly impossible to kill, and water loving. I took Mom these in substitution and told her they were immune to the privacy curtain. Saying that line with a straight face took some effort, but she believed me without question. I prayed over the health of those plants regularly on my visits, but they did remarkably well. At one point, someone gave her a Christmas cactus, and after a few months, she became concerned that it was not in a pot like the others. She thought it needed a pot *precisely* like the one her healthy pink plant was in. This came up months after I had bought and potted the pink plant, and I had a time trying to duplicate it. I finally found something nearly the same size, shape, and design, and that sufficed.

She went through a phase of believing that there was an extraterrestrial warlock who visited her in her room. It took her a while to work this out, she reported, because he was invisible, which is why nobody else ever saw him. She finally realized his presence because she saw things moving about her room on their own. I had to wonder if the whole story was designed to explain visual and then auditory hallucinations. Once she figured out that the warlock was behind this, it was all okay, and she began having regular conversations with him. She wasn't in the least afraid of him and assured me that "he's a *Christian* warlock and a gentleman." She said he was interesting to talk to. Eventually, he proposed marriage and started building a house for her. As the Director of Nursing said once, "She can have the most logical, focused conversation on something imaginary that I've ever heard."

There were also at times delusions of being under attack, much like the ones out at Erdenheim during the bad summer. She would sometimes sit down by the nurses' station, drawing safety in company, and then once they found her huddled in the back of her closet. All we could do was try reassurance, Ativan, and, if the threats persisted, yet again tweaking the psych meds. It was horrible seeing her so scared.

Then there were the wheelchair racers. Mom often would sport a bang or bruise on some body part throughout her life, and this held true and later increased at the nursing home. She hurt herself there, often with witnesses, in exactly the same way she had hurt herself in her functional life; she simply got too focused on a direction she was heading and failed to adequately adjust to miss an obstacle in the way. But to explain these bruises, she told me that people held wheelchair races in the hall and kept banging into her. She had complained, but since they never did it in front of anybody else, no one believed her or took any action against them.

Mom started clawing at herself—scratching is too mild a word—and literally had long, raking, bleeding wounds on her arms or her ankles at times. We tried everything, including investigating for a physical problem. The laundry tried changing soap. There was no rash, and her actions never had the appearance of someone scratching an itch. It wasn't the constant, nagging annoyance of itchy skin. Sometimes she wouldn't do it for days or weeks, and then she would spend a whole evening at it with nothing new in her routine that particular day. You could ask her if she itched or hurt or was uncomfortable at all, and she would say no while clawing at herself. They tried lotion. They tried medicated creams. They tried scrapings and lab tests to see if something turned up.

They even made an appointment in the city with a dermatologist for a specialist's opinion, and I drove down to be present. She rode the nursing home van up from her little town, and we met at his office. He was polite, thorough, and sympathetic; I remember the silent squeeze that he gave my arm as he was leaving the room. Mom was fairly alert and answered his questions, but all of her answers carried the same theme that she had no problems, nothing was wrong, and she didn't scratch herself at all. Other people did this to her. He prescribed a new cream to soothe her skin, but he said that in his professional opinion, the problem was mental. Unfortunately, I agreed. It would have been easier to treat a physical diagnosis. He did suggest Ativan p.r.n. at the bad times, which she was already getting, and an antihistamine, though not Benadryl, which can react badly with demented patients.

I remember that that day when we left the dermatologist's office, I pushed her to the waiting nursing home van, but when the driver put down the wheelchair lift at the back, Mom didn't want to get on. She wasn't throwing a fit, but she was hanging on to me, always asking another question, refusing to let the aide take hold of the chair handles. Finally, I got onto the lift myself, rode it up into the van with her, and talked to her for a few more minutes while she was being strapped into place. I then left her with a promise that I would visit her soon, and she accepted that.

Two other delusions came up about this time that were related, I think, to the skin difficulties. One of these involved the "pepper girls." Mom said that girls would come up laughing when no one was looking. These girls would pepper Mom's wheelchair or her clothes. They even started using "meltable" pepper that would be invisible when anyone was looking for it and would then reconstitute itself after the chair/clothes had been certified pepper free. Mom began to take napkins to "vaccinate" against the pepper and stuffed them down the sides of her chair as well as in the seat, which she said was the only thing that helped. She fussed that nobody would believe her and make them stop, but one day, she told me that after lots of prayer, she had concluded that the mature Christian thing to do was to turn their behavior over to God and rely on his ultimate justice. I promptly agreed that that was a very praiseworthy attitude to take and that God would fix everything in the end.

She also decided abruptly that she could only wear pure cotton. Not only that, she insisted that throughout her life she had always worn only cotton, which wasn't true. This came up during a call one day, one of the times when she insisted on talking to me and the staff put through the call for her because they couldn't settle her down. That conversation was painful. She said that I had brought her down a bunch of new clothes recently, which wasn't the case, and that they were not cotton. "I know you had good intentions," she said, "but you don't understand." She had never been able to wear anything else all her life, and I had messed it up. The whole phone call involved her assuring me that she knew I had brought everything noncotton or mixed material down there in a well-intended mistake.

I was scrambling at first to figure out what the problem was, because she was in mid-delusion, and I had missed the front end of that one. Once I realized what she believed, I told her that I would make an extra visit down, that we would sort out every last piece of clothing she had, and that she could approve or disapprove it. I also said I'd look for a few pure cotton things if I could find any to buy and bring her. She was satisfied with that and closed the conversation with, "And remember, we wear the same size, so it's easy to buy for me. We wear the same shoe size, too. Size nine." Both of those facts were entirely correct. I was left wondering as I hung up how it was possible to be so out of touch with reality and with memory and yet still recall that we both wore size nine shoes.

One of the most painful delusions involved her deciding she had had a baby stolen from her. She was looking for this baby and trying to get someone to help her. Being presented with a doll did no good. Being told others were taking care of the baby and the situation and that the child had been found and was safe never helped. She would actually dissolve into tears at times worrying about this kidnapped baby and wondering why the world wouldn't listen to her. "I suppose they don't believe me because I've never had one before," she told me several times. "But I *did* have one now, and it's been taken." Referring to the labeled picture on the wall of her with her four children and counting to prove all were doing fine didn't help, either.

Not being able to help: those were the worst days. To the end, she still recognized me most of the time.

There were days when she didn't, but those weren't the days that broke my heart the most. I had long since been convinced through prayer that I was doing what I was supposed to, that my sole assignment right now with Mom was to be there for her. Not to do anything; there was nothing left to do. Just continue *being* there. But she wanted me to do something.

There were days she was ready for me to take her home right then, and home was always Erdenheim. Even when she could no longer say the name, the description was unmistakable. This was never some long-ago residence or childhood memory. She wanted the farm. Many times, she asked why I had kicked her off to have it to myself and told me, "I wouldn't have bothered you." There were other days she would want me to solve this or that or intervene with the staff and get them to make the pepper girls or the employee of the month stop persecuting her. Worst, there were the days when she seemed to want me to fix her mind and make the illness go away.

Over the years I sometimes took classical music selections for us to listen to together. It was never her beloved Rachmaninoff now; the composer is too gifted at incorporating the full spectrum of emotions. No, what I took for Mom these days was unfailingly soothing, pieces by Bach, where everything always makes perfect sense, or Brahms' "How Lovely Is Thy Dwelling Place," which is a musical hug wrapping securely around the listener.

On my own, however, I started listening more often to Rachmaninoff's *Prelude in C-Sharp Minor*, and increasingly, the piece seemed to illustrate the course of her illness to me. The opening chords, firm, solemn, like bells tolling, but still with almost a gentleness to them in the echo—those were the initial symptoms, the memory loss slowly gathering momentum. Then the abrupt plunge into that middle section, musical rapids in a river of sound, turbulent, agitated—that was where we were at this point in her life. The sudden dive into it would have been February 22, 2008, and the current course with all its twists and turns was perfectly accompanied by the music.

The piece isn't long, and no matter how busy I was or if I was driving and had reached my destination, I always kept listening until the end. In the final section, it returns to the solemn theme of the opening, slowly getting softer, and then, at the last, come those two ultimate upturned chords. Mom had loved that lift at the end. That would be the final phase of her illness, agitation resolving again into a peaceful sadness, a "solemn joy," softer, and then lifting at the very end. Always, of course, the piece brought me not only sadness and beauty and recognition but also humor; that echo of "FISH FEATHERS!!!" was still ringing.

Mom was moved back to the locked unit in spring 2014, having tried again to escape a few times, and she was getting much worse functionally, too, even starting to lose the ability to maintain conversation. She still had clear words at that point, but she no longer had fluent conversation. Her reading also had stopped by then. After she was back on the locked unit, there were many visits when she refused to let me leave, when she would be paddle-rolling after me or trying to hang on to me. Sometimes staff could distract her, sometimes not, and if parked in another room, she would be following me even before I turned around.

Several times, I had to run away from her at the end to leave. I would turn her one direction in the hall, take her to the end opposite the unit doors, then whip around and sprint for the exit, knowing she couldn't turn herself around and then match my speed down the corridor. I only did this as a last resort on days when all else had failed, but I never was able to do it without turning back for a last look as I keyed the code to let myself out. She would be coming down the hall after me and looking straight at me with the most hurt expression in her eyes. If a staff member had her, even attempting to point another direction or go into another room, she would fight her way into turning around and still would watch my escape; she could be amazingly strong physically. I hated those days.

I took Tenuto down several times over the years, and her bedside manner was always exemplary. The last feline visitor, however, wasn't Tenuto. In autumn 2015, I decided to take Pharaoh, a kitten I had acquired from a home aide client. I'd started working with the home health agency again part time in early 2015, and the client I had the most hours with was Cat Lady, who had thirteen cats already and then had another litter dumped on her that summer. Pharaoh was the runt of that litter, and I had taken Pharaoh home with me once the kitten was old enough, Cat Lady insisting that since I had named that one, that one was mine. Pharaoh—jet black and silky once healthy—was calm as kittens come and had a sense of humor, and I thought this cat might work for a visit with Mom. I intended to test Pharaoh as a possible therapy cat to alternate with Tenuto, but when I got there, Mom was phasing in and out of orientation. When she was in, she loved the kitten, stroking and commenting on the fur as Pharaoh purred up a storm. At other times, not even the cat in her arms seemed to reach her.

That, I decided, was it. Oddly, while I could handle Mom not recognizing me at all and simply put those days down to the disease, I didn't want to see her not recognize the presence of a cat. It may sound crazy, but that was how I felt. I simply couldn't handle seeing a cat mean nothing to her. I decided to make that day the last feline visit, to leave it with still some positive moments, even if intermittently. It wasn't planned out that way, but somehow, it seemed appropriate that Mom, the lifelong defender of stray and down-on-their-luck street cats, had the last live cat she held be not the purebred Siamese Tenuto but a dumped, rescued waif of unknown heritage that was now blossoming under love.

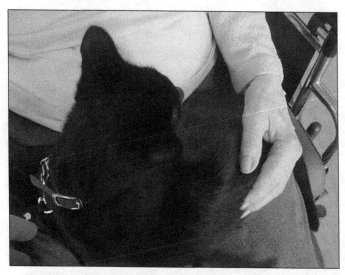

**Pharaoh in Mom's lap on the last feline visit.**

The disease continued but waited, as if the world were holding its breath. I was reminded of a favorite poet of both of ours, Coleridge, who once said, "Day after day, day after day, we stuck, nor breath, nor motion, as idle as a painted ship upon a painted ocean."[20]

That was how it often seemed over the years. Life was paused, even though the roller coaster with its crises, hills, and even an occasional loop-de-loop kept rolling on. Everything had changed, but nothing ever did now. I knew, of course, that each day drew her closer to glory, that this was *not* how the rest of existence for either her or for me would be, but sometimes, it seemed that I had spent twenty lifetimes driving back and forth to the nursing home, going in, watching her mental collapse, and then doing it yet again a few days later. We seemed stuck in an event-filled, delusional way of life.

It was in 2015 that the thought first struck me as I drove home from a visit that both of her parents had lived well into their eighties. That realization hit so hard that I had to pull over for a few minutes, lost in prayer. *No, God. Please, no.* Mom had now entered her seventies. She could not, I could not, *we* could not take another ten to fifteen years of this. *Please, Lord, have mercy.*

It was one of the rare prayers to which you get an instant sense of answer. I wasn't given a time frame, but I was convinced and reassured that no, there wasn't another decade and more on this seemingly endless road. And for what there was left, strength would be provided, even if it seemed at times like the tank was near empty.

"If I forget, yet God remembers."

I put the car back in gear and drove on, but while Robert Browning's beautiful words were yet again, for the hundredth time, running on one mental track, another one offered up the prayer from the end of Revelation.

"Even so, come, Lord Jesus."[21]

# 14.

## *Diamonds*

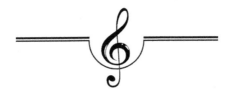

They never failed to surprise me. In the midst of the turmoil, sometimes even on quite bad days, there would come a sudden gleam of light, lasting only for seconds. For one brief, precious moment, there would be a diamond visible glittering amidst the coal. Throughout Mom's long illness, they occurred, not every day or month but often enough that it would recharge me a little and also provide a precious memory to hold onto, a memory of *Mom*, not of her disease.

This happened not just with Mom. I didn't visit Grandmother and Granddaddy nearly as often as she and Vicki did, and I'm sure I missed several, but there were also such moments with them. One Christmas, we were waiting in the library for Vicki to arrive to start the family celebration. Grandmother was near the end of her life, a pathetic, crumpled doll in her wheelchair, only the lap buddy holding her up. We had brought down a tape player and had put on highlights from *Messiah*; Mom always insisted on *Messiah* at Christmas gatherings. The Hallelujah Chorus started off, and Grandmother, who hadn't spoken in months, perked up and started singing along, accurately, taking the alto part; she had always been an alto. Mom and I stared at her and at each other, then joined on soprano, and for nearly a minute, the three of us sang together. Then Grandmother faded out like a radio losing the signal and was gone again. "She's rehearsing for the heavenly choir," Mom said.

"That was neat," I agreed, "but we probably don't have to rehearse in heaven."

Mom shook her head. "I agree, but can you imagine her accepting that?"

No. Grandmother, the hyperperfectionist who wanted every single thing straight always before she set foot outside the house, would definitely feel as though she should rehearse for the heavenly choir, whether or not it was necessary.

A diamond.

One diamond with Granddaddy was the prayers. To the end of his life, he could pray, even when he couldn't hold a conversation. The staff remarked on that. Still the old preacher ("pastors never retire," he had often said), he could offer a totally coherent prayer for the food or someone sick or whatever else was needed even from the middle of confusion. Just ask Granddaddy to pray for something, and he first would take off his hat. He loved hats and often wore them even indoors, but not once in his life, I think, even with Alzheimer's, did he forget to remove it to pray. Then he would give himself completely to the requested prayer for that moment. After the amen, orientation usually left once again, but for those seconds, he was himself, not merely reciting words but truly offering thanks, concern, or whatever was appropriate to the situation. They say that with dementia, things you have done most in life are the last ones to be forgotten. Granddaddy must have spent much of his life in prayer.

For Mom, that charge down the ramp, followed by her neat stop at the bottom, was a diamond. It was frightening to watch, but ever after, I think, the word "Whee!" will remind me of Mom on the ramp at the nursing home. It was a glimpse of her old joyful passion for life peeping through the dementia. Watching her, I could well believe that as a toddler, she had ridden that galloping horse and loved every minute of it.

One day, I had come down for an extra visit. Mom was in a very agitated spell just then, and I was playing some of her beloved classical music in an effort to calm her. Right in the middle of fretting about being persecuted and the actions of her current employee of the month, she paused and said, "That's a lovely glissando," and her hands swept an imaginary keyboard in front of her, giving life to the word. A moment later, she reverted to her complaint, but I now remember her tone, her expression, and the reach of her hands whenever I hear one in music. Glissando. A diamond.

She could pop out occasionally with vocabulary words like that even after her mind was failing so much that her usual conversation was on a far lower level. A few years before Mom's death, James and Beth adopted three children. They did get to meet Mom a couple of times when they came down to visit; I'm glad she had the chance to see her new grandchildren. But the day I was telling Mom about the upcoming adoption, I reported the children's names, which all happened to start with A. She tilted her head and said in the old familiar tone, just as if we had once again been discussing poetry together, "That's nice alliteration." Alliteration. Another word with an extra shine to it now.

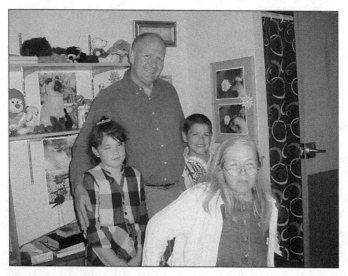

**James with two of his new children visiting Mom.**

Then there was the day well into her illness, after her transfer back to the locked unit for the second and final time, that she told me she had received a spoken message from heaven. She brought it up about five times that day, but she never could hold the thought long enough to convey what the message was. She didn't seem upset, just forgetful, but in fishing and trying to prompt her, since this obviously meant so much to her that visit, I asked if it had been a bad message or a good one. She looked at me in surprise and said, perfectly clearly, "Nothing bad comes from heaven." True, that.

She used to fuss at herself for forgetting things, and there again, she sounded exactly like her old self. All her life, Mom had talked to herself, to the furniture, to the cars, to the animals, and to anything else that was handy. The years fell away when I heard her fumble for a word or the end of a sentence and then abruptly switch out of confusion and say with all the old tone, "Now, Paulette, you know what you mean. Get your act together!" It was a glimmer of Mom whole, reminding me that she was still in there, even if mostly buried by the disease at this stage of progression.

One similar Mom-of-yesteryear moment came during another visit when I asked her as usual if she had had a good week. She said yes, she had had a good week, and everything was okay. Then the expression changed for just a moment, the clouds fell away from her face, and she looked around surreptitiously and said to me with her old smile, "She says with trepidation."

Early in 2014, there came a diamond I wasn't there for, but the staff told me about it later. A resident on the unit was passing away, and her whole family was there to see her off. They had stepped out into the hall while the nurse was doing something, and they huddled up and were praying. Mom was roll-pacing the hall in her wheelchair as she did so often, and she spied their huddle, rolled up to them, sang a hymn fairly well on tune, and then rolled off. It was even an appropriate hymn, I was told, though the staff member couldn't remember which one.

Michael's next-to-last visit to Mom also came in early 2014. He came into the room and said hi to her, and Mom reached out and grabbed his hand. She clasped his hand the entire visit so tightly that he was afraid it might be hurting her, but she wouldn't ever lighten up or let go. That day, she knew him and knew that seeing him was a rare treat. I'm glad Michael got that diamond to hold onto through the upcoming years; his last visit in 2016 would be a much harder one.

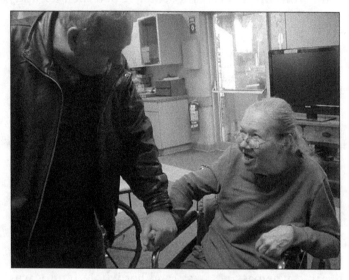

**Michael with Mom in 2014.**

At Christmas 2014, with Mom well into very advanced illness, I was singing carols to her. Mom by that point had mostly lost her singing. I hated to see that go; music had meant so much to her her whole life, but she couldn't remember words or tunes reliably anymore. I was singing "Hark, the Herald Angels Sing," and Mom suddenly chimed in on alto.

It was her singing alto that got to me especially. Mom was a soprano, although she could go very low in range for one, as could I. That was one reason our occasional part-swapping trick had worked so well on former duets over the years. But when we weren't part-swapping and were simply singing a straight duet, or for the highest parts of songs where we were part-swapping, she would sing alto to my soprano, because I had two more notes on top. When simply singing to herself or in a congregation, she always had automatically taken soprano; the only times in her life she had sung alto throughout a song as she did that day were when she was singing a duet with me. That's what made it a brighter diamond in December 2014. Mom wasn't just reacting to the song or momentarily remembering words and notes; she was singing a duet *with me* and knew that, and she responded appropriately and assigned herself the alto line, just as she would have in past healthy years.

Not every visit, but for the majority of them, Mom—if in any mood except pure agitation—would say to me as I left, "Thank you for coming." Sometimes even on days when I had to spend most of the conversation telling her why she couldn't come back home with me to Erdenheim. Sometimes even on days full of stolen babies or Christian warlocks or beauty shop ladies with evil scissors. I can hear it in her voice now, and I heard it literally hundreds of times over her nursing home years. "Thank you for coming."

In late May 2016, about two months before her death, I was visiting one day when Mom was very restless. She kept trying to climb off the recliner they had her in, so I was physically blocking her in and singing to try to calm her down. She kept chiming in, just a few notes here and there. By that point, this didn't often happen anymore, but she did it that day two or three times, so I pulled out the phone in an effort to share this diamond with the family.

"Can you do it for the others?" I asked. She was mumbling some nonsensical word salad as I started singing. "This is my story. This is my song, praising my Savior all the day long." The mumbling died away, and Mom joined in with me, speech garbled, tune not totally on pitch, but unmistakably there as she sang along on the repeated phrase. "This is my story. This is my song, praising my Savior all the day long."[22] The moment safely captured, I put the phone away, and later that afternoon, I sent it to all the family along with the weekly update. It was the last video ever taken of her. I still pull it out at times to watch it, and I'm sure the others do, too. I look at her expression as I listen. She was not just reciting words and notes. Her face lit up, and her eyes focused a little. She was praising still.

Diamonds.

# 15.

## *Humor*

There were other moments, not diamonds but episodes when I abruptly would be trying, and sometimes failing, to keep from laughing. Some of what she said and did during her illness was absolutely hilarious. The depth of the fall remained tragic, but those inserts of humor, like the diamonds, could catch me by surprise and brighten a dark day. Her tone and reactions could be so much *her*, even if the content was badly confused.

Mom wouldn't have minded me laughing at times. She always placed a very high value on a sense of humor and described it as an essential survival skill in life. There were several times in dealing with her parents' illness when she laughed at something they had said or done.

She absolutely loved Judge Judy. Never having had much time to spend watching TV in her working life, she made up for that in the nursing home, and Judge Judy was her favorite program. "She doesn't put up with nonsense," Mom noted approvingly. However, as the confusion increased, she had no concept of schedules or channels. She truly expected the TV obediently to follow her wishes no matter the time of day. Early one year, in the midst of the football season where even I as a nonfan kept hearing about This Bowl or That Bowl, I came into Mom's room at the nursing home to find her fuming. There had never been any doubt in her life when Mom was fuming; the sound effects and practically the smoke hung around her like a cloud.

"What's wrong?" I asked.

She smacked a hand against the side of the TV. "Football, football, football. All that's on is *football*! Don't they know that I want to watch Judge Judy?" Mom, the lifelong hater of sports, was genuinely annoyed, unable to understand why the TV channels insisted on showing this silly stuff when anybody would prefer Judge Judy instead.

I actually sent that story to Judge Judy, emailing it to her website, and I received a reply a few days later that she had read it and was amused. So was I. Every time now that the season of This Bowl and That Bowl is upon us, I remember with a smile Mom and her frustration with the TV schedule.

Another sports moment took place a few years later, with the confusion scale still higher. I arrived for a visit and found Mom up in the sun room watching a baseball game on the large screen TV. This in itself was proof positive that she had lost it, as Mom would not have sat still and watched anything-ball in her prime voluntarily while she had the ability to leave. At the least, she would have been crocheting or such while waiting for the band at halftime rather than paying attention. This day, however, she was definitely watching the baseball game, and she was laughing as if it were one of the funniest comedies she had ever seen. I greeted her and inquired what was so funny, and she answered, "Those silly, silly men! They keep running and jumping and waving and falling down, and then they just get up and do it all over again. They can't decide what they want to do." A nearby aide and I both dissolved into laughter on the spot. Baseball in a nutshell as described by the demented.

Her imagination to the end remained remarkably active, even if confused. One Mother's Day, all of the female residents were given a rose by the facility, but Mom was somehow convinced that she alone had received one, and she was trying to figure out why it had appeared. Her explanations for this were remarkably varied. She had a secret admirer, the florist had lost the delivery card and misdelivered someone else's, and even the Rose Fairy ("You know, like the Tooth Fairy") had been making rounds.

Another day, I arrived to find her looking morose. I asked what was the matter, and she said she was so very sorry about Mrs. Claus. Mrs. Claus? You know, Mrs. Claus, Santa's wife. I asked if something had happened to Mrs. Claus, and she said yes, she had died, and Santa was grieving. This conversation took place in late summer, and I made a comment to the effect that Santa soon would have work to plunge himself into, as it wasn't that many months until Christmas. Yes, Mom replied, he was aware of that, but he was also worried about her flowers. She had all sorts of flower beds, and it was now his responsibility to take care of them. I couldn't resist pointing out that Santa lived at the North Pole, hardly prime real estate for flower beds, and she gave me her well-known "don't be ridiculous" look and said, "I *know* that. Of course, they're *inside* flower beds. Mrs. Claus even had an inside sun made for them, because it gets dark so long up there, you know."

One day when she was still in the general population before her final transfer back to the locked unit, I had come down to eat lunch with her. She was full of paranoid fears that day, looking under the tablecloth, and then she started to tell me what the ice-cream machine did—and it wasn't that it made ice cream. In midsuspicion, she got distracted by something and switched channels, as she could do so quickly at times. Meanwhile, I was left wondering the true purpose of the ice-cream machine. I even tried to cue her back into that delusion over lunch just to satisfy my curiosity but to no avail; she had completely changed topics. Several of her delusions were recurring, but that one appeared only that day and then was gone forever. I was glad she had stopped being bothered by it, but part of me also felt like you do when you discover the last page of a book missing. To this day, I sometimes wonder what exactly that ice-cream machine did.

When Nik Wallenda, the tightrope daredevil, walked across the Grand Canyon, I reported this to Mom at the next visit as a harmless but interesting piece of news. "Hey, Mom, this last week, somebody actually walked a tightrope across the Grand Canyon."

Mom looked at me with all her old expression and replied in all her old tone, "I'll bet he was a man."

On a similar note, there was one day well into her illness when I arrived to find her watching a TV program on wrestling alligators. Her comment: "That's an insane job. I thought some of mine were tough, but that's truly crazy." Yes, Mom, I agree.

Speaking of TV, the staff once in a care plan meeting got to talking about the viewing preferences of the residents on the locked dementia unit. They enjoyed older Disney, though did not like the newer; in particular, *Frozen* was a total failure with the audience wandering away during showings. Their favorite two things to watch per the workers were *Shrek*, which they never got tired of, and, surprisingly, *Shark Week*. They were mesmerized by *Shark Week*, not scared but rapt.

Mom's imagination worked overtime again regarding the plane ride to heaven. She told me one day that she had received yet another message, and this one was that she was going to be dying soon, but because "I've been here so long, I can't go the normal way." So her trip to heaven was going to be a five-hour ride in a plane. They were making sure that all details were covered for her trip, including arranging quotas on luggage and asking if she got airsick. I was smiling listening to this, and Mom concluded with, "So good-bye if the plane happens to come before I see you again." I objected that I wasn't going to tell her good-bye, because no matter when she went to heaven, I would see her again. She nodded in satisfaction and said that was right, then returned to details of packing and snacks on the flight. She even actually packed a few times, and her choices there were ludicrous. One day, for instance, she picked up a pillowcase, inserted a stuffed cat, one shoe, and a napkin, and pronounced herself all ready for travel.

She talked to her stuffed cats as if they were real and even told me a few times that she had to be sure to pet them all equally, lest some get jealous. One day in her last year, I brought her a new stuffed tiger, and I took a few pictures of her with it. She objected that those weren't good pictures and that "I have to get him settled first." I told her to set him up as she wished, then, and she tried out several wacky positions and finally wound up with his nose in her stomach and his tail up in the air. "There," she said, "that will be a perfect picture." I dutifully took it, and she was satisfied.

When Cat Lady, my main client on the home aide job, died near the end of 2015, I told Mom about this on the next visit, including the fact that Cat Lady had had sixteen cats, and while I managed to rehome a few, I wound up installing most of them outside as barn cats at Erdenheim. She considered this solemnly, then said with respect, "That's a *lot* of cats." I reminded her that she certainly could have rivaled me on cat collecting during her life, and she laughed herself and added, "At least we don't have mice." This exchange came at a point where she rarely put two coherent and connected sentences together into a conversation anymore. While feeding out at the farm I sometimes hear it again in her tone: "That's a *lot* of cats." Yes, Mom, but you still have me beat for the family record.

Then there was the day not many months before the end when I arrived to find the residents still finishing eating. They must have started late that day; by then, I tried not to get there while they were at meals, but this time, they were still working on dessert. Mom was in her place up at the feeding table with the residents who must be fed each spoonful and couldn't eat on their own, so there were several staff members sitting right there. I came up beside her, gave her a hug and said hello, then noticed a bruise on her thumb, obviously her latest casualty from rolling straight into things. I asked, just making conversation, "What did you do to your thumb?"

Mom raised it and studied it as if she had never seen it before, turning it to survey all angles. Then she looked back to me and said absolutely clearly and seriously, "It came that way." The staff at the table cracked up as quickly as I did.

Even in the depths, some days, I still could find myself laughing. Wonderful gift of humor, threading black storm clouds with silver.

# 16.

# *Crafts and Breaking Patterns*

Mom always loved crafts. In typical Mom fashion, she sometimes bit off more than she could chew, but also in typical Mom fashion, she plunged on nevertheless to complete things—perhaps not perfectly, but it always got done. There was only one exception to that I can recall in her crafting life, and thereby hangs a tale, one decades in the making, starting back in her prime of life but delivering the punch line during her advanced illness.

In Mom's childhood years, Grandmother did try to interest her in sewing. Grandmother made many of her own clothes and did her best to impart this education to both of her daughters. Mom, however, never especially liked sewing. This might have been because the resultant product was clothes. Mom simply never was interested in clothes, and she and Grandmother had those early disagreements over spending her money on books and music rather than wanting a special new outfit.

Once away from Grandmother's house and on her own, Mom did make some clothes, and she always wanted to get into needlework, such as counted cross-stitch, embroidery, and yarn projects. The interest was there, but in dealing with three young children through her first marriage, she never had much time.

After we moved to Missouri following the fire, Mom decided that the time had come to expand her horizons. She bought a book on crocheting and a few simple cross-stitch kits and plunged full speed into learning those skills.

Around the same time, she noticed me watching her projects with fascination, and she gave me a crafts basket for my ninth birthday. I have it to this day, somewhat cat scratched now, but Mom would appreciate that addition. It stands on scissor legs, about two and a half feet high with the fabric basket about a foot deep suspended at the top. Mom prefilled it with all sorts of things: thread, plastic canvas, needles, yarn, a pin cushion, and more, including a good set of scissors. "Always remember, there is nothing like a good set of scissors."

So in the evenings, as Mom would craft for an hour or so whenever she could chisel the time out, I would likewise craft. In fact, with more spare time than she had, I did it more regularly. I can still hear her on those shared evenings talking to her work. Mom talked to *everything*. "No, no, no. I saw that thought. If I want you to drop, I'll tell you about it. You think you're going to make me lose count, don't you? Well, you're *wrong*. I have no intention of it."

She quickly discovered that counted cross-stitch was not her cup of tea. She admired the finished projects, but the absolute rigidity of pattern, the intense counting, and the need for every tiny stitch to be in the correct place grated on her. Her personality always had chaffed against tight restrictions. She finished a few little five by seven kits, but she didn't buy more. When I got into rug hooking, she studied it and came vicariously to the same conclusion: this was not for her.

Crocheting, however, was something she took to immediately and enjoyed. Her first project was an afghan for me. (Mom never started small, except with the cross-stitch kits—perhaps she was dubious about her tolerance for that from the first.) It took her over a year to finish the afghan between her job and her night classes at the university, but she kept plugging away at it, and she loved it, seeing the creation form beneath her fingers, even if while fighting a cat occasionally for possession of the yarn.

After my afghan was completed, she made one for James. Where mine had been pastel shell stitch, his was red, white, and blue ripple, very patriotic looking. Then came an afghan for Michael, orange and brown variegated with an eggshell white border. Last in line, she started one for herself. We both admired the yarn for that one, blue, green, and white variegated colors. I especially loved the pattern, and so did she. It was the most complex pattern that she had tried yet, one not in her book but that she had had someone recommend to her and write down. It made a beautiful textured effect. She did comment many times that it was much harder than the others, but she still enjoyed the work.

Then she met her second husband. There ended Mom's serious crafting attempts. From that point, she was caught up in her short second marriage, the arrival of my youngest brother, the divorce, and the total reshuffling of life, shortly followed by the beginning of her parents' illnesses and subsequently by the approaching shadow of her own. She set her afghan aside half finished in 1983, but she never got back to it, though she said she intended to.

Meanwhile, I kept crafting myself with the limited time available for it. Unlike Mom, I loved counted cross-stitch and made several family presents. I also enjoyed rug hooking, plastic canvas, crewel, and crocheting. I even carved her a cat out of wood once, a rough amateur effort at a cat but certainly recognizable as one. She named him Caricat, after caricature, pointing out that he was smiling.

It was in 1989 that I decided to crochet Mom a sweater for Christmas. I was away at college, providing convenient work time with her nowhere near, and I could use myself to try it on as it progressed, since we were the same size. The sweater was milk chocolate brown, and she absolutely loved it.

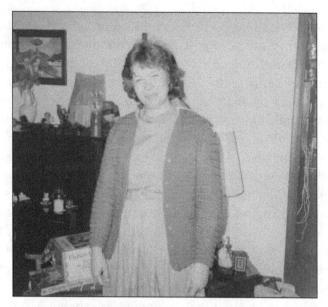

**Mom in the sweater I crocheted for her,
Christmas 1989.**

When she went to the nursing home, that sweater went along, and it became her Linus' blanket. She wore it almost constantly. The staff had to seize moments very strategically to wash it, because if Mom missed the presence of her sweater, she threw a fit. Always, she remembered that I had made it and would tell people that. As she progressively ran into things and caught it on corners going by, it became pulled out of shape and even developed a few holes. I was willing to let her happily destroy it, but one day when I came to visit, she declared that it needed to be retired. She gave it to me with full ceremony, asked me to take care of it and store it safely, and then, with a thoughtful look, contradicted herself. "No, give it away. It's old and worn, but surely there's somebody who doesn't have a sweater at all." Even in her advancing illness, her innate compassion remained. I didn't donate the sweater, of course. For one thing, I thought she might change her mind or forget her decision, though she never did. But I couldn't have discarded that. It wasn't wearable any longer, but it was tucked lovingly away with holes, pulled yarn, and all in Mom's own cedar chest, now mine.

The last thing I made for Mom was a very simple cross-stitch. She was progressively mixing up names, usually knowing me but getting very tangled at times in speaking of others. She had a picture of me on the wall beside her bed and one of James. James, the one of us who was into genealogy, had made a simple framed family tree for her with a picture of him with Mom on the page. Still, there was nothing to that point on her wall with all of us together in one shot.

For that last craft gift, I took one of the few pictures of all four of us kids with Mom. Given the wide age range, those occasions had been very rare; this one had been taken at Michael's wedding in 2005. I attached the picture to some counted cross-stitch fabric, then gave it a few roses around the edges. Across the bottom, I spelled it out in black thread carefully, Paulette Webb with her children, and I named us in order in the picture. That joined the gallery on the wall next to her bed, and I would go over us with her on visits.

The final unexpected craft project, a surprise joint effort with Mom, contained a delightfully unpredictable twist of the sort so typical of her personality. In going through her things after her placement in 2008, I found her half-finished afghan from the early 1980s, along with the remaining skeins of yarn. I was very glad to find the yarn, as we never would have matched the dye lot after all these decades. I decided to finish that afghan myself, making it half by her and half by me.

I never mentioned finding the afghan to Mom. At that point in 2008, just after her placement, she was very restless and unsettled, and I was afraid she'd ask for it and declare in an independence fit that she would finish it herself. Perhaps that was selfish of me, but the extant half in the box had been made by Mom whole, Mom in her prime. Her attempting in 2008 and after to add to that section would have frustrated her extremely. The stitch was too complicated for someone with dementia unless that person had far more crocheting miles on the odometer than Mom ever did; she had found it hard even in the early 1980s. She probably would have ended up destroying the thing, ripping out stitches in annoyance that they wouldn't work, maybe even "disciplining" it as she did the tape/CD players. I couldn't stand the thought of something made by her, something she had loved working on, now being torn up. No, I decided to withhold it for myself, and she would never miss it if she didn't know.

However, I couldn't find the pattern, that wonderful, fascinating pattern, the one she had said was so hard, the one not in her original book. No scrap of paper with written instructions remained in the box with the afghan and yarn. She had never mentioned the name of the friend who had given it to her. All of my efforts came to naught for quite a while on identifying that stitch. I looked in every book I could find, posted pictures on the Internet, and showed the afghan directly to a few very crafty folk I encountered over the years. Nothing.

Then one day around 2014, in the middle of Walmart, I found it. As I flipped through one of the little booklets of crochet stitches in the crafts section, a search I had made many times before, there it was. It was called basket weave. No question; this *was* the pattern for Mom's afghan.

I bought the booklet, came home and studied it, looked up a video on the Internet for confirmation that I understood, and then with relish rolled up my sleeves and pulled out that storage box. The project begun over thirty years previously, the one which would be made by both of us, finally was going to be completed. I started out—and within five minutes, I was laughing so hard I couldn't see straight.

The pattern is based on multiples of four. You do four (or eight or twelve or so on) stitches one way, then do four (or eight or twelve or so on) another way, then back to the first method, over and over again. It isn't as hard to count as those tiny little squares on counted cross-stitch, but you stay on your toes keeping track of your place. It is definitely a city traffic version of a craft stitch, not a highway driving version.

Mom obviously had started out with the best of intentions. The first rows were exact, and from that point, it began to slip. She always did have trouble with strictly defined systems. Instead of four, four, four, Mom had done four, six, four, three, four, four, four, two. Whether by conscious rebellion or unconscious chaffing at the rigidity of it or both, she had broken the pattern over and over. That was Mom. That in a nutshell was Mom. Her personality filled every stitch of that half afghan even more than I had realized. The funny thing was, it was barely noticeable. Not until you took a hard look and started counting the thing did you realize that it didn't count right.

The second half of this decades-delayed crafting joke hit me almost immediately after the first. While the afghan didn't look bad at all at this point, I couldn't possibly complete it according to the correct pattern. To have half of it crocheted by Mom's kinda, sorta, dancing-around method and the other half by the actual instructions to the letter would be obvious. The contrast side by side only would serve to underline the differences.

Unlike Mom, I can follow a pattern until the cows come home. I don't mind at all learning new patterns and even find the experience fun, but I want there to *be* a pattern. Randomness annoys me. Even when I was a child, randomness annoyed me. Now, to finish our joint project, I was going to have to deliberately break the instructions. Furthermore, I would have to do it inconsistently, careful not to let myself define a new pattern and simply follow that one for the next hundred rows.

Finishing that afghan was a joy. Her presence permeated it. As I crocheted away, forcing myself to miscount, I wondered sometimes which of us the joke was on. Was it Mom, trapped by her own stubbornness and choice into a project that required her to stick at least in the vicinity of a strictly defined system? Or was it me, forced by memories and, yes, stubbornness, if I wanted to make it match, to let a pattern slip and be more flexible?

Either way or both, God has an awesome sense of humor.

# 17.

# *"Does She Still Remember You?"*

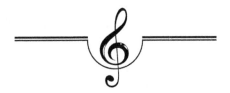

O ver and over during Mom's illness, I would be at church or a music rehearsal or some other gathering, and the question would come as somebody asked about Mom. "Does she still remember you?"

I solemnly swear never to ask anybody that question for the rest of my life.

There are a few reasons that question became grating over the course of the years. First, there was the sheer frequency. If twenty people asked me a question about Mom, nineteen of them would ask that one. It was by far the leading question in a runaway victory, leaving all other contenders in the dust. I heard it literally hundreds of times. At a gathering, it was quite possible to be asked well over a dozen times in the course of two hours. Of course, it was an expression of sympathy and support; I do realize that, and I appreciated the thoughts. Still, by the time the fifteenth person there asked me, it was wearing thin.

Questions, even well-intended ones, can become a burden if repeated constantly. A well-known Christian comedian posted on Facebook that after her husband died, she was ready to snap by the time the fiftieth person in the visitation line asked her how she was doing. I remember an occasion in choir rehearsal at church, after a member's husband died, when her daughter said that her mother should be back at church the next Sunday and then made a plea: "Please don't ask her how she's doing. Everybody has been asking her that, and when it keeps coming over and over, it gets overwhelming."

There's also the fact that a question requires an answer. That may seem obvious, but I myself had never thought it through to realize that if a person is exhausted and near the limit, already dealing with a long-term situation, repeatedly having to give an answer to a question on the spot can rob some of those precious remaining ounces of energy. Not until Mom's illness did that come home to me so strongly. There were days when putting one foot in front of another was my goal for the next hour, and having seven people in that hour want an answer right then was difficult. I'm sure I have done exactly the same thing unknowingly in the past, but I am going to try to be more aware in the future.

Then there was the fact that probably seventy-five percent of the people who asked me if Mom still remembered me followed it up with the statement, "When they can't remember you, that's the worst thing." Not a question but a declaration, leaving no room for doubt that that was indeed the worst thing.

Only it wasn't. For me, it wasn't. Thus an intended expression of sympathy and camaraderie actually drew a bit of added distance between the speaker's experience and mine. I'm sure from the frequency of that comment that it is indeed the worst thing for many people, but people's reactions do differ, even within the same family when you really are talking about the same situation. No two individuals respond identically in absolutely every single respect to a stressor; as Mom often said in reference to people, "God loves variety."

When Michael visited Mom for the last time in the spring of 2016, she did not know him. That hit him hard that day. I don't know if it was the worst thing in her illness for him, but it probably was in the top handful. Dad and Rena visited Mom roughly four times a year throughout the nursing home era, and he usually would comment in those later years as we drove away, "She didn't know me."

Maybe it was the fact that I saw all of Mom's course firsthand for the whole seventeen years, riding on the same roller coaster car in the seat directly behind hers, but there were several days I wound up dreading more than the blank look of unrecognition as I walked in the door. She had a very protracted, difficult course, and from February 2008 on, declining memory was never her worst problem. The staff and the doctors themselves commented many times on that. She also was not steady in her course, not a slow spiral down. Her peaks and valleys were steep ones. Today was not a predictor of tomorrow in mood or mental stability, and what she knew or didn't know today might not apply the next.

Did she still remember me? To the end of her life, the answer was most of the time. There were plenty of days that she didn't. I do know what it was like to walk in and have a lengthy conversation with her and realize that throughout the entire time, there was no clue in this person's mind who I was, that my own mother, who bore me and raised me, had no memory at all of the relationship.

But worse than those, at least for me, were the days when she would be hallucinating or delusional and terrified by something, and I would try to soothe her with only limited success. How do you convince someone that the room is not on fire, that the refrigerator is not possessed, that people aren't attacking her, or that there isn't a baby lost out there needing her help?

Forget distraction; though I always tried that, Mom could hang on to things like a bulldog sometimes, in that way reminding me of her former self before her illness. Tenacity was one of her greatest strengths in life and also at times her greatest weakness because she would carry it too far, which she herself freely admitted to me. After she got sick, with the fear and demented confusion added to her vivid imagination, many days became a living nightmare for her. Nor could you convince her that the situation was being dealt with by others, so she didn't need to worry about it. To her mind, she had to address this imaginary crisis herself, and she knew at some level that she was no longer capable of handling it, and that terrified her. I hated watching her go through those moments.

Then there were the several times when she knew full well who I was and would ask me why I had kicked her off Erdenheim to have it for myself. "I wouldn't have bothered you," she would say in tears. "I knew it was your farm." Other times, she figuratively and occasionally literally had her bags packed when I arrived and was ready to leave the nursing home that moment, had just been waiting for my arrival to get her, and I would have to explain yet again that she couldn't leave.

There was more than one visit when I entered the nursing home and a worker would say as I walked by, "Good luck." I would sigh and steel myself, and I knew already on those days even before seeing Mom that the problem wasn't going to be that she didn't recognize me.

The days I had to run away from her to be able to leave. The look of pure hurt in her eyes as I turned back for a moment at the security door after sprinting down the hallway and saw her rolling after me at her best speed. Those days were heartrending.

But those still weren't the worst thing.

What was the worst thing, at least for me? It was the days when she wanted me to fix it, not just an individual annoyance, like the pepper girls or employee of the month, but the entire illness. She would remember sometimes that I loved to organize and sort things out, and she would inflate my ability and expand it to areas far beyond my control. While I hit my limits back in 2008, to her, some days, I had no limits, and she would not just want but expect me to turn the world right side up again and make everything, including her mind, the way it used to be. Not able to comprehend or admit her illness in the later stages, she still knew that something was seriously wrong, that all of life was disrupted, and she would turn to me for resolution.

On those days, I would enter her room for a visit, and she would look at me with clear recognition, no doubt at all who I was, give a bright smile, and say, "Ah, sanity!" That word will have negative associations for me for the remainder of my mentally intact life. My heart would drop to my shoes, and I would send up an arrow prayer. Once, I even pulled out my cell phone on the spot and shot off a one-word text to Rena: "Pray!"

Sanity. What that word meant to Mom was, "Here comes my daughter, who can sort it out and fix whatever this big thing wrong with all of life is, and everything will be all right again."

Then I would sit down, and she would ask me, in different rambling, demented ways but usually coming down to the same confident words at the end of her complaint. "You can fix it." I would try gently to distract her or at least settle her down, knowing that I couldn't give her what she wanted and so trustingly expected of me. The growing hurt and disappointment in her eyes were like a physical blow.

That, for me, was the worst thing. I would far rather have had her not recognize me on a visit than have a "sanity" day requiring one of those conversations.

What made it bearable? People and their prayers. Music many times. Above all, the certainty that Jesus *did* understand, that he knew as nobody else could exactly what I was feeling every moment. He knew the worst thing and all the other horrible things and the tiredness and stress and the humor and the diamonds. All of it was shared. On the days when she didn't know me and also on the days when she did and merely forgot my limits and expected the impossible, I could almost feel a heavenly hug at times and the reassurance again that, "If I forget, yet God remembers."

I always did realize the concern and sympathy behind that question from people. While the question itself became overwhelming by the end, I would try to reframe it into other words mentally, knowing that what they really were saying was, "I'm thinking of your mother." The thoughts were appreciated, and the person making an effort to express those thoughts, not just leaving it in silence but making me aware, was appreciated even more.

Which words helped the most? It wasn't any specific "formula," and I can't speak for others, but what helped me, at least, the most out in public were simple expressions of sympathy with no question attached, no demand for an immediate answer on the spot, just letting me know they were there. "I'm thinking of you." "I'm praying for your mother." "I often think of your mother and remember her in choir." "I think of her when we play the hand bells; she loved those so." "Still remembering your mother in my prayers." If I had the energy and time right then, I usually would respond with a brief update on her status, but I appreciated the fact that I didn't feel pressured to by the perpetual question.

The youth pastor at the church once went down to visit Mom and afterward sent me a sympathy card, one of those intended to be used after a death. He reported the visit, that he had told her he was from church, and that he would keep praying for the situation. Those prayers and the fact that it was a sympathy card and not just a blank "any occasion" card conveyed his message perfectly. That card was a balm across the day. I kept it and reread it. I still have it.

A few other members of the congregation during her illness sent cards with various Mom memories from back in her prime. Sometimes people also would mention those moments to me in conversation when we met. Most of them had known her for years and years, and she was definitely memorable. I always enjoyed the old stories and learned some new ones.

The church was there throughout her illness. I never once doubted that, and it made a lot of difference. The prayers of people around me, however expressed, helped carry me through those seemingly endless years.

# 18.

# *Falling*

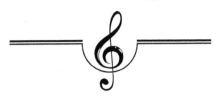

Mom started falling more.

She had fallen occasionally throughout her nursing home stay. She had even fallen a few times back when she lived on Erdenheim. However, starting around the end of 2014, the frequency climbed sharply. Almost all falls were caused by the same thing, getting up and attempting to walk off. Her balance was so shaky by that point that she couldn't walk off, but not remembering that, she still would try. She also never remembered to set the brakes on her wheelchair before standing.

The staff diligently did their best, but we ran into two major complications in handling Mom's increasing falls: Mom's speed and a set of government regulations, which themselves seemed to me to be demented.

Mom's speed was unbelievable. You had to see it to fully grasp it; she could launch out of that wheelchair like a grasshopper. I have been standing within two feet of her myself and still missed preventing a fall and could only control it somewhat when she decided it was time to rise. There was often no prelude or warning on her part; she would just flip abruptly from peacefully sitting to standing up in one second flat. The staff told me that they worried more about her than anyone else on the floor (all others also demented) in terms of falls because she was so fast that you couldn't do anything to prevent it unless you had your hands directly on her already before she took a notion to get up.

Grandmother had fallen a few times, too, back in her day, once even breaking a hip. After that worst one, the nursing home simply used a lap buddy, a foam rubber cushion that fit between her stomach and the front bars of the wheelchair and held her in. Problem solved. This, however, wasn't permitted any longer by Mom's era because of new regulations. Patients, even blatantly incompetent and unsafe patients, could not be "restrained." No lap buddy, no seat belt, no obstruction of any sort to their freedom of motion. "They have the right to fall," more than one worker told me with exasperated helplessness. The staff hated that rule and its effects as much as I did.

That regulation had me grinding my teeth in frustration on many a day. I do understand that elder abuse can occur and also recognize the possible temptation for convenience restraint just to keep people out of the staff's hair. Still, you would think that some standards of determination could be reached in high-risk cases, such as a patient meeting the following A, B, and C criteria of dementia and prior fall history. No. Nothing that restrained a patient's physical movement was allowed any longer in the nursing home setting. Someone behind a desk somewhere who didn't even know Mom's name and didn't have to see the growing catalog of bruises and injuries we did had decided that they knew what was best for her better than we, her caretakers.

The staff tried what they could to help. They moved Mom's room down to the one directly opposite the double doors into the common/dining room where the big TV was and where most patients gathered at all hours of the day. That patient room across the hall was easiest for anyone working in the big room to see into and monitor, even while busy with other patients. They wrapped her wheelchair brakes with hot pink tape to try to attract her attention. They used a stand-up alarm for a time, but again, Mom was so fast that the warning wouldn't give them time to get there before she took a tumble. They switched her wheelchair for a while to a reclining model. Briefly, that helped, but then Mom started getting agitated at her inability to paddle pace, and when she fell out of that one while trying to get up, she would climb it and fall over the sides, resulting in worse falls than the simple stand-up-straight variety. They sent her to occupational therapy for several sessions trying to drill safety steps in before they gave it up. She truly was unable to retain any instruction.

Of course, they tried medicating her. She was on Ativan around the clock now with extra p.r.n. for especially restless periods, and they did try other sedatives instead in case she just didn't respond best to Ativan any longer. They also tried to adjust and find the perfect balancing act on her antipsychotics and other dementia meds. The problem, as ever throughout her nursing home stay, was that her response to medication wasn't always consistent. What was perfect today could fail tomorrow, then be fine again the day after that. More and more often, in terms of her physical abruptness, the medicines were starting to fail.

It was a nightmare of mine that she would break a hip. She never did, though we had a few close calls, even once requiring portable X-rays in the nursing home, but I was terrified that she was going to. By this point, the nursing home was her security blanket, her familiar environment. Moving out to a hospital would have been very hard on her, kicking off a whole new string of fears and delusions and hallucinations. She would have wound up restrained very quickly there, which was still permitted in hospitals with combative patients. The thought of having her tied up, totally disoriented, frightened, and unable to be settled down even if I had stayed around the clock throughout her stay, which I would have, was my greatest fear the last few years of her life. I even had it written in the front of her chart that she was not to be transported out of the facility to a hospital in the event of illness, but of course, in the case of an injury like a broken hip, which was causing acute pain and could be quickly fixed with a procedure, I would have made an exception.

I prayed daily that she not break a hip, and that prayer was answered. I also started around the same time praying more diligently about a wish I'd already had in mind. I wanted to be with Mom when she died, present at the actual moment. Given my two jobs and the fact that she was an hour and a half away, this could be difficult, especially if death came quickly at the end. Still, I wanted to be there, and I petitioned for that regularly. The desire recalled all the years of shared music, of our playful duets, of her singing on every occasion around the house as she lived and worked, of her singing in the hall in the four-story house after we young children had gone to bed, the song finding its way unerringly through each child's open door. Music had meant so much to her at every point of her life. I wanted, if possible, to sing her to sleep.

In addition to falling, Mom seemed to lose all sense of obstacles in her path. This had nothing to do with vision; as well as we could, both the staff and I checked that. She could see fine, but she seemed to have a total lack of interpretation of what she saw at times. This wasn't a failure of peripheral vision but of what was right at eye level straight ahead. She would roll the wheelchair directly into a wall or a door or a counter even while looking right at it, then say, "Ouch," in surprise. She would also roll straight into and over people. This wasn't at all intentional; she just continued with her paddle pacing on a straight line once pointed in a direction until she hit something or someone that forcibly changed her course, like a wheelchair-bound pinball trapped in a diseased game. The other residents on the locked unit, all of whom were themselves demented, even came to realize and retain this. The path parted in front of Mom like the Red Sea, with patients dodging right and left to get out of her way.

Of course, the upshot to both the increasing falls and the running into barriers was that she was one constant bruise or abrasion. That last year, she always had an injury of some sort somewhere.

There were other less physically painful failings that became evident. Her speech gradually grew garbled, with fewer and fewer intelligible words. Speech had been so far ahead of functionality for most of her course; it was this that enabled her so fiercely to defend and protect her deficits and to appear normal in conversation for a few minutes. Back at the neuro-psych testing in March 2008, when she was scoring down to the 0.02nd percentile and even lower on the performance scales, she still ranked extremely high, far above the standard population verbally, and the doctor had commented then on this unusually wide discrepancy.

During that last year, she also developed a new habit that everybody around her remarked on. She started singing to herself. There was no recogniz-able tune or words, and volume was pianissimo. Still, there was no doubt that was what she was doing. Mom had always sung throughout her life on all occasions; the difference here was that it was so obviously pri-vate, just for her, no longer overflowing exuberantly to the world around. This wasn't due to any lack of lung power. She could still achieve plenty of volume vocally when she wished, but the self-singing was always soft, quiet, intimate.

Her singing in prior years, even on contemplative pieces or soft lullabies to the children, had carried a force and power and transmission. When the only audi-ence was herself and God, if anything, she had enjoyed even more singing full throttle, holding nothing back, and more than once when driving, she had attracted the attention of the police by her speed, which had unconsciously increased with the momentum of the music. She also on those occasions, with typical Mom forthrightness, had admitted that she was singing and got carried away, and the police accepted the excuse and just gave a warning. But singing with focus turned inward instead of outward was new for her.

I tried a few times to join her or to tease the unknown song out into the open, and she would look at me blankly. Asked what she had been singing, she would seem puzzled and say, as near as I could tell, that she didn't know she had been. She could still be prompted into singing aloud rarely if I worked at it, but those occasions were always with a song I started. The private self-singing was hers alone. She had never done it before that last year. She did it multiple times a day from that point until a few weeks before the end.

At the care plan meeting in the fall of 2015, the brief cognitive screens that they routinely did on all patients had declined to a new low. As the social worker put it, the only way she could have scored lower at this point would have been if she were dead. On no measure could they get anything any longer from her. It was at this meeting that they first brought up hospice.

I turned it down then, but a few days later, I received a call from the Director of Nursing asking me why I didn't want hospice. She was very polite and matter of fact, just asking my reasons, not challenging the decision. I told her that the sole reason was the "within six months of death" technical definition I had heard. I thought Mom, with her infamous stubbornness, still had longer than six months to go, and I was afraid of running out the funding and being left with nothing to help us. I knew she was dying, just didn't think we were quite that close yet.

The DON informed me that six months is a very loose guideline, not a rigid rule. As long as people continue to get worse, and neither of us anticipated Mom doing anything else, they can stay on hospice. She knew of people who had been on hospice for a few years. She guaranteed that hitting the limit wouldn't be a problem if we went past six months, and she also said, a statement I didn't appreciate fully until later, that it could "make some things easier" at the end. Mom was already on full nursing home care, so the words puzzled me. Still, the DON strongly recommended hospice at this point, so with the timing concerns put to rest, I agreed, picking the hospice associated with the aide agency I already worked for part time. Neither the DON nor the hospice let any grass grow under their feet. Within five minutes of my hanging up from that call, the hospice called me. We arranged to meet at the nursing home the next morning, where they would screen Mom.

Mom's screening didn't involve much of her personally. She mumble-answered a few questions, or at least responded to being spoken to, then rolled away in the middle of her own sentence after five minutes. The hospice intake coordinator went through her chart and talked to me for over an hour, explaining everything and confirming the DON's statement that as long as you were getting worse, you couldn't run out of hospice. The nursing home staff would still provide most of Mom's care, but the hospice team would be supplementing that with bath aide, nurse, social worker, chaplain, and music therapist.

Hospice also would be in charge of medications now, and that was the major change we discussed that morning. They wanted to delete everything deletable. I said that the antipsychotics and the Ativan were absolutely necessary; Mom at her unmedicated worst could tend toward violence. Those, I was assured, would be left alone. The focus was more on dropping maintenance drugs, such as for her hypertension or the multivitamin. Keeping her healthy was no longer the goal; that ship had sailed. Comfort and manage-ability were everything now. They also wanted to stop Aricept, pointing out that it was intended to slow the effects of Alzheimer's, and that ship also had already sailed. I agreed on the condition that if she reacted negatively to deleting it, we could add it back. She never did. Mom's remaining course, while still a roller coaster, wasn't any more of one than it had been with the additional medicines.

Mom enjoyed hospice, I think. She loved the music, talked on good days with the chaplain and the social worker, and the nurse and bath aide visits were also extra attention and care. Everyone was careful to keep me informed at each step. The social worker and the chaplain both called me right at the beginning to ask for details on her, things that she liked, and ways that she responded best so that they could tailor their encounters to her personality.

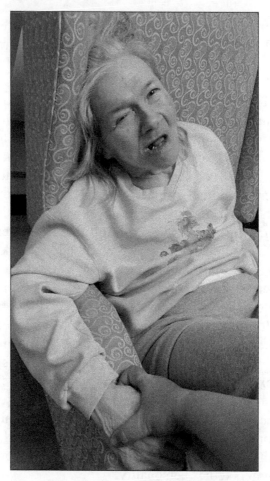

**Mom in the last year of her life.**

The falls continued and remained our biggest worry. There was no fractured hip but a seemingly endless list of bruises, abrasions, and lacerations. The staff tried to watch her as closely as they could, and over and over, we would stress wheelchair safety to her and try to tell her it was because we didn't want her to fall.

That brief flare of Mom's old personality would pop out there sometimes as she would reply, "I have no intention of it."

I kept the cell phone on and with me all the time, but the one place I would turn the ringer off was in church right before the service. That led to one memorable morning. I checked the phone right before going into the choir loft, but when the choir left the loft after our anthem that morning and I looked at the phone quickly in the back hall, there was a missed call from the nursing home. Caught up in the anthem, I hadn't felt the phone vibrate. There was no good reason for the nursing home to call me on a Sunday morning when the staff all knew perfectly well that they would see me in a few hours anyway.

However, that morning, I was going to be singing the solo. I didn't have time for more than a quick drink of water in the back hall before reentering the sanctuary. I couldn't return the call right then. So I went back in and sang, and that morning, the song was "The Majesty and Glory of Your Name." It had been one of Mom's favorites, too, both as a choir anthem and as a solo; I have a recording of her singing it. That morning, the glorious words and soaring melody were even more of a prayer than usual to me. It was one of the hardest solos I've ever sung in my life, not knowing what was going on right then, just knowing that something was. After I was done, I slipped back out and called the Manor, and of course, Mom had fallen again. Thankfully no broken hip, but she had banged up and cut herself.

Mercy. More and more, I was running out of specific words to pray about Mom, and it consisted mainly of looking mutely at God in appeal. Always, I prayed

that she would be protected in the falls, and I prayed
that I would be there when she died to sing her to sleep,
but beyond those two requests, I was getting to the point
where all the words just distilled to one heaven-directed
plea: have mercy. I had no doubt still that the prayers
were being heard, but I no longer prayed them in words,
just the whole spirit extending hands upward. *Lord,
have mercy.*

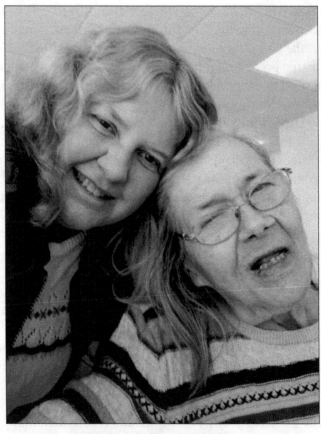

**Me and Mom in 2016.**

Michael visited in May 2016. He had not seen Mom in a couple of years, and the jolt was extreme. No weekly updates could fully convey the decline. Mom was actually having a quite good day that day for her current status—calm, responsive, and interactive in a confused way. But to him, it hit hard. She didn't know him, and much of her speech couldn't be understood. As we sat around the table, I saw Michael's wife, Melanie, the nurse, studying Mom, the professional assessment obviously rolling along silently, and I was glad she was there to help talk to him later. We all knew that he would never see Mom again in this life.

At the end of June, Mom had a very bad fall, banging her head and face severely. The hospice nurse had been there, and she called me while I was on an aide shift. Of course, all my aide clients knew what was going on. I had explained to them why I would take calls from the nursing home or the hospice, even if working right then, and they all understood. They were even concerned and prayed about Mom themselves. After such calls, they would ask, "Is she all right?" Of course, all of us knew she wasn't all right, but the sympathy was appreciated. One of my clients once even sent Mom a little stuffed cat she had found at a garage sale for a quarter.

On my visit a few days after that fall, I took a picture of Mom all battered up. I had been taking more pictures of her the last several months and attaching them to the weekly updates to try to give family a visual as well as verbal report of decline. This one I remember titling, "Mom emulating Rocky."

Then, just as she was getting past acute bruising into broader and more colorful beginning-to-heal bruising, she fell again and once again hit her head. This time, she hit it against an edge and sustained a couple-of-inch gash on the back of her scalp. The staff stopped the bleeding, butterflied it together, and called again to report.

July 6, 2016. This was the fourth specific date that was seared into my memory of Mom's illness. February 22, 2008: the day the power company crisis began and we stepped out of simple memory loss into all the rest of it. September 16, 2008: placement. April 9, 2009: Mom's sixty-fifth birthday, the day on which I signed the papers transferring her out of the nursing home to the full-scale psychiatric hospital. July 6, 2016: the date of that last care plan meeting and the decision made there.

There would be one more date that joined that list a few weeks later.

On July 6, I went down in midweek for a care plan meeting. Mom had had her second bad fall with head injury just the day before, and as I entered, the Manor nurse was in the hall and called me aside. She said, "She's really hurting today. I think the two bad falls so close together hit her hard. I called to request some Roxanol to give her for a few days until she starts feeling better." I nodded my agreement and went on up to the unit first, before the meeting, to see Mom.

She was pathetic. Her entire forehead was green and yellow, remnants of that first fall, and the gash on the back of her head from the second, while neatly cleaned and treated and pulled together, was impressive. Worse than that, though, were her eyes. She was hurting, and she was scared. She didn't understand what was happening in her world anymore, and on that day, for her, there was only pain. I talked to her, and she perked up enough for some conversation. I sang to her for a little bit, and then I left her to go down to the care plan meeting, filled with new resolve that we *had* to figure out some strategy to stop the falls.

Falling, of course, was the main topic of the meeting. Mom otherwise seemed stable. She was too thin, but her weight had been steady for the last few months. The various department heads and I sat around the table trying to brainstorm anything to do about the falls. No seat belt, no lap buddy, no restraints in her wheelchair due to the regulations. Again, we discussed the reclining wheelchair they had used for a while, but they agreed that that had backfired in the end. Mom's continual roll-pacing was impossible in that, and when she had become agitated at the forced stillness and tried to climb out, she had sustained worse falls than from the regular chair.

As we hit a silence for a moment, all staring help-lessly at the roadblock, I cast my mind around desper-ately for anything else that we hadn't tried yet, and I remembered the nurse's comment on my way in that day. Roxanol. Liquid oral morphine. Enough of it would slow down anybody.

"Could we start using narcotics full time?" I asked. "Not just p.r.n. like we have before but around the clock and in larger doses. Enough to slow her down physi-cally. Maybe then she *couldn't* decide to get up and then fall, and I do think she's in pain."

The staff looked at one another. "I know it can cause dependence," I said, "and I know there are side effects, but does it matter as much at this point? She's really hurting herself now."

The social worker spoke up. "I think some of these patients who have multiple falls do have pain contributing to their restlessness."

"She's got to be hurting anyway," another staff member said. "As often as she bangs herself up. I've heard her say ouch."

"I've heard her say ouch, too," I agreed. That had been when she rolled straight into something, not as a general comment, but still, she was one constant bruise or cut these days. She couldn't be comfortable physically.

They agreed to put in a request with the hospice to go to round-the-clock narcotics, and there we left it. Nobody else could think of any other option. We had already run through all others, and any lesser medicating of her had also failed to stop the falls.

After leaving that meeting, as I walked back along the hall that ran perpendicular to the ramp from the upper levels, including the locked unit, I stopped there at the T intersection and looked up that ramp. I remembered her rolling down that ramp, pushing off from the top and calling, "Whee!" on the exciting descent, then reveling in her neat, tidy stop at the bottom. I couldn't see the unit from where I stood, but I knew Mom was up there. She would have hated being drugged up, but she would have hated all of this by now. After a moment, I walked on. I regretted the necessity of the decision, but I was at peace with it. There was nothing else left to try, and she was truly hurting herself now.

*Lord, have mercy.*

# 19.

# *"Like a Solemn Joy"*

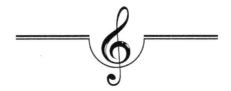

As always, the hospice was promptly efficient, and I received a call from them fairly soon after that care plan meeting. This was from the hospice nurse, who first verified that, as requested by the nursing home, I wanted to start using narcotics in larger doses and full time. After I confirmed that, she covered the requisite fine print, though she didn't linger on it.

"We can do that," she said first of all. "It's not a problem. But I do need to make sure that you realize that there can be side effects to these medications. It could impact her level of consciousness, and it could affect her appetite. They also are respiratory depressants and suppress breathing. This could shorten the remainder of her life."

"I know," I replied. I had known that already back in the care plan meeting at the moment I'd asked. That wasn't my reason for the decision; I only wanted to stop the increasing falls and injuries, and we had already tried and failed with everything short of this step that I could think of. Still, I did realize what was quite likely to happen.

The nurse accepted the statement and then said that she agreed that Mom was in pain by now from her constant falls. In fact, she even wondered on the latest exam this day, a few days after her second bad head injury fall, whether Mom had done something to her left leg in that fall. It was in the thigh, toward the knee, and she seemed more sensitive to touch over that leg now and to hurt whenever it was moved. No point in diagnostics; they would change nothing on our plan of care. In any case, the nurse said that she agreed that going to heavy-duty painkillers full time was appropriate at this point.

She continued with specific plans. "We have this all approved. We're going to place her on a fentanyl patch and also use Roxanol every four hours. That should make her comfortable now. We can start it today." It suddenly occurred to me at that point that medication issues were probably one of the things to which the Director of Nursing at the Manor had referred when she told me months before that hospice would "make some things easier." Probably without hospice status already in place, there would be more of a process required to change to a heavy-gun narcotic regimen like this.

I agreed to the plan, and the nurse promised regular updates and hung up. I had received that call while driving, and I watched the miles going by as the car sped on, wondering what mile marker Mom was passing. Was this the beginning of the acute end, nearing the exit? It could well be. Her life was still ultimately in God's hands. I just hoped that whatever happened, her grasshopper jumps out of that wheelchair and the constant falls would stop. She was hurting herself too much at this point to allow it to continue.

In that much, we were successful. Mom never fell again.

It didn't take long for the other effects of the med change to appear. Mom's appetite completely vanished. That was going to be especially hard to deal with, because Mom had been adamant about receiving no artificial nutrition of any sort, not even IV supplements. The idea of being fed by other means during a chronic illness had revolted her; she'd often said she'd rather die. All those statements dated back to well before the onset of her dementia. Her wishes were clear, and I would honor them; if she stopped eating by mouth, then this was indeed the end.

Two and a half weeks. It took two and a half weeks after we changed the meds. Calls from the hospice personnel increased. Mom was also less responsive in general, though you still could get interaction from her at times. She did seem comfortable, at least. The hospice nurse increased visits in rapid succession over that time from three to four to seven days a week. I made extra visits myself.

We never stopped trying to get her to eat; the staff was diligent about it. She simply would not most of the time. I even took her a chocolate milkshake once. She wouldn't take the straw, and if some was put in her mouth, she would not swallow. She had been thin anyway, but more weight absolutely fell off during those weeks.

At a regular Sunday visit after church at the start of that last week, the nursing home nurse hooked my arm as I walked down the hall toward the unit. "You're within days," she said frankly. Then, with a smile, she added, "More and more the last week, I think she looks like Ivy." Ivy was Mom's mother. So many employees who had worked at that facility with Grandmother and Granddaddy years ago were still there—blessed, caring people who still remembered faces from days long past because all the faces truly were people, not merely patients, to them.

I thanked the nurse again for all they had done, and then I repeated, "I want to be there. I know it might not happen, but if it can, I'd appreciate you letting me know when you think we're down to hours."

I went on up the ramp, along the hall, and through the locked doors onto the unit. Mom was in bed, and I saw the difference immediately on that day. She was looking at heaven, seeing the gates swing open. There was an otherworldliness to her expression, and she was smiling, not at me but at the visions of glory.

I sat down next to her and started talking, trying to imagine her release. "You're going to sing in a choir again," I told her. "Imagine the music of heaven. You wondered what Bach and David would have written with all these centuries to work on it. You're about to find out soon."

She did know I was there, but conversation that day was one sided—almost. Right at the end, as I was about to leave, I said, "I love you," and she promptly and clearly replied, "I love you, too." Those were the last earthly words I would hear her speak.

On Monday, the hospice called and said that she had started running a fever, which apparently is quite common as someone nears their final days. On Wednesday, when I came to visit, Mom looked all but dead already. Sunday, she had looked transported. Wednesday, she looked awful, so bad that I concluded that I wouldn't take any more pictures of her, not even for the family updates. She was near comatose with occasional quiver twitches, and twice as I stood there, she had a full-scale seizure. I stayed and watched and held her hand until she came out of it. I didn't call for the staff; there was no treatment to be done, anyway. We were purely on a countdown by this point.

The social worker from the hospice arrived while I was there, and we talked for a while. She shared some of her memories of Mom over the months: her love of music, her attempts at courtesy even from confusion, her sweet spirit. The worker and I sang a few hymns, and while Mom hadn't spoken or opened her eyes this time, I thought she was registering me, not just the music but me. Just as I was thinking it, the social worker commented, "She knows you're here. She's paying attention to you."

After the social worker left, I stood there having a debate with myself for a few minutes. Based on everything I was seeing, she looked as though she might die in the next thirty seconds, but my gut feeling was, "Not quite yet." After some consideration, I decided not to stay. I did go into the sun room and ask one of the staff for a pair of scissors, a closely guarded treasure, of course, on that floor of dementia. With those, I cut a lock of Mom's beautiful silver hair and took it with me as I left.

That night, Vicki went to visit Mom after work. She reported that Mom was awake and speaking to her, but she also said she estimated her weight now down to eighty-five pounds. That guess pretty well matched mine. "I hate seeing her like this," Vicki said.

Friday, I was planning to go visit Mom again after my morning aide shift, but I called that morning on the drive to the shift for the usual daily update. The aide on the floor said that she had been about to call me, that Mom's breathing was quite different today. She recommended that I come on. I pulled the car over on an exit ramp and then notified in sequence my aide client, whom I wouldn't after all be seeing in twenty minutes, all of the family, and both of my employers. Then I drove on, wondering if this would be the last trip down this familiar road. (It wasn't. Even after death, details remain to be dealt with.)

Mom looked much the same as Wednesday, already halfway through death's door, but there were two major differences. The quiver jerks from Wednesday were gone, and her breathing was irregular in a repeated pattern of quick, labored breathing for about ten seconds, then holding her breath for fifty-five seconds. Throughout that long day and subsequent night, I timed these intervals over and over against my watch. Time and again, I thought she actually *had* died during one of those pauses. I wasn't the only one; the staff themselves wondered it aloud a few times. Her eyes were closed, and she seemed unconscious.

I sent off a few quick text updates to the family. Rena replied, "Just stay there...you will most likely get your chance to sing her home."

Yes. Today, I would stay here. I had no doubt that this right now was the end, though Mom's stubbornness would wind up making an appearance as it so often did through her life.

I sang a few hymns to her, and then, realizing that this was probably going to be a few hours at least, I looked around for a chair. The visitor's chair was a few feet away, and I let go of Mom's hand so I could take those steps to retrieve it. As I released the pressure, Mom abruptly tightened up, gripping back, refusing to let me go. No words, no look, but there was for just a second strength and also recognition in her fingers. She did know I was there. Realizing that would help me in the long upcoming day and night.

"I'm not going anywhere," I told her. "I'm right here. I'm just getting a chair." She didn't hang on when I moved away the second time. I pulled the chair over, sat back down, and took her hand again.

Songs and prayers mixed. I had picked up my car book on the way in. (Lesson from Mom: always have a book with you at all times.) However, I don't think I read two pages in the whole twenty hours that stretched ahead of me. I was either singing to her or praying or looking up symptoms on the Internet on my phone and trying to plug them into a death timeline.

The staff was absolutely wonderful. They kept checking on Mom, turning her every two hours to prevent sores, swabbing her mouth with a sponge stick to try to alleviate some of the dryness, putting ointment in her eyes for the same reason. One of them even brought in a small dish of ice cream at one point, still trying even today to get her to eat. Mom would not swallow.

They also checked on me several times, and they brought me lunch and later supper. The bath aide from hospice came by and gave Mom a bath, and later, the hospice nurse arrived. She assured me that even though she herself was off tomorrow, another hospice nurse would come if Mom were still alive.

At one point in the afternoon, an aide from the nursing home came in. "I need to say goodbye because I'm off all weekend." Then she got right up to the bed with Mom, on the other side from where I held her hand, and she gave her a strong hug and said, "Goodbye, Paulette. I love you." She had tears in her eyes as she turned away.

Another aide told me, "I know we aren't supposed to have favorites, but she is one of mine." Then, with a smile, she added, "My favorite was the aliens." Mom definitely had added imagination to her dementia.

I also heard the full story from one of the aides of that final bad fall a few weeks ago, the one that had prompted the decision to change meds. The aide reported that Mom had been restless that morning. They had given her extra Ativan, and then while waiting for it to kick in, since she wanted to get up and walk so badly, they walked her up and down the hall between two of them several laps. Finally, she was out of breath and complained that she was tired. They then settled her back in her wheelchair. Mom said she was just going to rest for a while, that she was worn out, and she really did look it.

The two staff members made sure she was comfortable, then turned away and started to walk off. "We didn't get ten feet away before we heard her go down," the aide told me. "I couldn't believe it. She was perfectly settled in that wheelchair, and she was still out of breath and saying she was tired and needed to rest. I couldn't believe she jumped up that quickly right then." I told her it wasn't her fault. I had seen Mom in action myself, and she could indeed change from peaceful rest to trying to stand with unbelievable speed. I know they did the best they were allowed by the regulations to keep her safe.

God bless you, nursing home workers.

In early afternoon, Mom was moved down the hall to an empty room because her roommate was getting agitated at all the activity, even though they were trying to keep the roommate occupied in the sun room. The staff carefully moved not only Mom but also the chair I had been using and the little cart of snacks and drinks they had brought me. I took along Mom's favorite stuffed tiger and put it in the bed with her, not quite dying with an official cat purring at you but as close as I could get. The room we wound up in turned out to be Mom's old room before her move up to the one at the end of the hall opposite the sun room doors. Now it was barren, unoccupied, impersonal. I sat there remembering the dozens of visits in this room, and I sang and prayed and timed periods of no breathing.

Vicki had called at one point and promised to come by after work. It was nearly 8:00 before she got there, which had me amused. All her life, Vicki was notorious for being late to family meetings. She brought along her daughter, Jennifer, Jennifer's husband, Caleb, and the latest baby, only a few months old.

We discussed Mom's condition first of all, but then they asked about my car, having noticed it in the parking lot. Kipling had been totaled in an accident about a month earlier when a man ran into me on the interstate, and while the insurance claim was still trudging through channels, I had acquired Frost, another Focus.

Frost would be the first car of my life in which Mom never took a ride.

We also discussed timing on the funeral. James, Beth, and the recently adopted kids had a family vacation scheduled for the next week, and while I'm sure they would have changed plans, I saw no reason to disrupt their trip. Mom's death was hardly coming as a surprise; they might as well use the reservations they already had. Michael also was playing into the estimated funeral timing. He had the farthest journey and also in his taxi driving schedule often had good days for work around the weekend. Putting those two different situations together, I estimated Wednesday in a week and a half for the funeral, and Vicki and company agreed that it was as good a target as any.

Vicki asked me if I was going to stay, and I replied yes. I would stay for the whole night if it came to that. She didn't think Mom was quite that close herself. "Mother held on for almost a week when she looked like that. It could still be days and days." I remembered that Grandmother had hung on beyond all medical explanation, but I still felt myself that Mom was close, quite close now.

After about thirty minutes, they left, needing to get the baby home. Vicki said she could come back at some point on Saturday if needed. Before they departed, Caleb asked me if I would mind him giving a prayer, which of course I didn't. He voiced a wonderful prayer for Mom's peace, comfort, and safe journey if death was the outcome here, as it seemed to be.

Then they left, and it was Mom and I once again. I sang and counted breaths, sang and counted breaths. Darkness had totally fallen. The sounds of the nursing home gradually hushed and stilled, and night gripped us. I watched Mom and remembered, remembered so many things from over the years, backwards to the beginning with my childhood, then forward through the music and adulthood and living and working with her for so long, then through the illness. It was finally over, I realized. The sickness was all but over now. Heaven was waiting; the door was open. All she had to do was take that step through it.

Once again, as so often over the past years of dementia, Robert Browning's incredible words played in my memory and soothed me. The music and poetry took over, expressing it all. The darkness outside, the circle of light in the room. The waiting. The upcoming farewell, both looked forward to and grieved over. The end, for now. Mom's life in this world was over. "If I forget, yet God remembers...I know thee, who has kept my path and made light for me in the darkness, tempering sorrow so that it reached me like a solemn joy."

# 20.

# *"Take My Hand, Precious Lord"*

The night wore on, and I was wearing down. Those incredibly long gaps between breathing spells continued but never seemed to vary, timed over and over again right around fifty-five seconds, and Vicki's words that Mom might go on a week like this replayed in my mind. It seemed impossible. No, every sense I had confirmed for me that the end was very close, but I couldn't decide what I was basing that on. Nothing indeed had changed for hours and hours.

By morning, I would be totally fried and would have to have a sanity and sleep break, I knew. Still, I hated to leave her. I wanted to be there, had prayed to be there. The months-old wish was as strong as ever. I wanted to sing her to sleep, as she had sung us to sleep so often long ago. Of course, God might will it otherwise. Mom might even be waiting for me to leave. I had heard stories of people who had hung on until one specific relative arrived or who, conversely, waited for a moment when the watchers had stepped out, as if not wanting to burden them more than necessary.

That thought hurt, honestly. If Mom wanted me gone, part of me could understand, and I would deal with it if she died five minutes after I left tomorrow, but the idea still hurt. I wanted her to accept this final vigil. We had been together through the whole seventeen-year road, and she had told me many times on the good days and in the more cognizant moments that she realized that and appreciated it. Of course, as I always replied to her, she had been there for us children much longer than that. A lifetime. Yes, it had been a good lifetime, full of love, adventure, pain, joy, and music. She had made mistakes along the way as all of us do, but there was never any doubt that she had loved her children with everything in her.

I alternated singing to her and talking to her as I sat there, and I kept my hand always on her arm. The nurse and the night aide came in regularly to check on us. The aide brought me another Diet Coke. She offered coffee once, having made a fresh pot, and I appreciated the gesture, but I had never been a coffee drinker.

Unlike Mom. Every thought tonight circled unerringly back to her.

The nurse checked her heartbeat again with the stethoscope, the only way it could be detected anymore. There were no pulses. The pulse oximeter to register the oxygen level in the blood wasn't giving any reading at all. The nurse said, "I wish I could get a reading. I'd wondered if she would be more comfortable with oxygen, but then again, it probably wouldn't do anything. You have to be breathing enough for supplemental nasal oxygen to help."

We watched Mom, who wasn't breathing again. The pause stretched out, knocking at eternity. I hadn't been timing this one, but the nurse and I both looked at our watches with the same thought simultaneously, that thought I'd had a hundred times already this last day and night. Was this it?

No. Mom resumed breathing, those awful breaths that she threw her whole torso and neck into. It looked horrible, but it looked no worse than it had several hours ago. Everything seemed on hold. Could she in fact keep this up a week?

I asked the nurse. "I know you can't give a definite answer, but you've seen a lot. On your gut feeling, is she right at the edge, or do we have more time?"

She gave me the favor of not repeating the disclaimer I had already assigned. "I think she's getting close."

I settled back for more waiting. "Just keep the pain medicine up," I said.

The nurse nodded. Then she left, and I sat there looking at Mom. She looked dead already. I waited for another spasm of breathing, then checked my watch when she stopped and when she started again. The same.

"What are you fighting this for?" I asked her. "Don't you know what God wants to give you? Just let go and accept it." A second later, the thought struck that God probably says that all the time about us, his wayward children, and I had to smile. Mom, like most of humanity and even more than most of humanity, was stubborn.

I sang her another hymn, then paused for a drink. I got up to get another cookie off the hospitality cart. Unlike that first moment Friday morning when I had moved away, she did not tighten her fingers on my hand this time. She hadn't for quite a while now. So some things in this interminable day were changing, were progressing.

My eyes drifted shut momentarily a few times, more with weariness, not dozing. I counted the breath gaps. Fifty-five seconds. I looked around the room. This was her former room; now it was empty, bare, waiting. I wondered if that new resident brought into here had died or had moved on to other arrangements. I wondered how many people over the years had died in this room. I wondered how long it would be until another name was added to that list.

Something was different. I snapped to weary attention, the conclusion preceding by several seconds the realization of what had produced it. Mom wasn't breathing again, but that was familiar. Yet *something* had changed. I studied her more closely.

She started breathing again, and this time, I spotted the difference. She was breathing longer. All day and night for hours, it had been ten seconds of breaths, fifty-five seconds of nothing. This time, she tried to breathe for a greater period. I waited for her to stop, then timed out the gap and the subsequent breaths. Twenty seconds of gap, twenty seconds of breathing.

I wasn't sure what the significance of that was, but after timing it through a few rounds, I stood up and stuck my head out the door to call the aide.

The aide came in quickly, and we both watched Mom. Fifteen seconds of gap, twenty-five seconds of breathing. "Does that mean anything?" I asked.

"I'll ask my nurse," she said. She left again, and I stood there watching and waiting until the nurse came.

"To me," she said after a moment of observation, "it says that she might be having some pain. I'll give her a boost on the morphine." She worked efficiently, measuring out the drops and, as she had all night, talking to Mom before administering them, letting her know they were coming, even though Mom wasn't reacting to us. But maybe she could hear. The nurse then rewet the cloth across Mom's forehead to ease the fever and wiped her mouth out with another cloth, trying to get a little moisture in for comfort without making it too much and choking her again. Mom seemed to settle a little, the breathing starting to flip back around, longer gaps, shorter efforts. We both watched her for a few minutes until she had resumed her former pattern, and then the nurse left us alone together again.

I sat down and timed it out. Ten seconds of breathing, fifty-five seconds of gap. Maybe it was just pain that had caused that brief inversion.

In the next moment, and for the first time since I had arrived Friday morning, Mom's eyes abruptly opened. I stood up and spoke to her, but she wasn't looking at me. She was seeing *something*; they weren't just blank. But it wasn't me. Mom's blue-gray eyes all her life had been certain giveaways to her mood and her physical status, and right now, they looked unutterably tired, more tired than I had ever seen them.

I started singing again, the first favorite of hers that came to mind, "Take My Hand, Precious Lord."

Halfway through, her eyes closed again. She stopped breathing, and then, as I was finishing a repeat of the song, sticking to the first verse for the words of it, she started up again. Ten seconds of breathing. Then it stopped, the same pattern yet again. The weight of seventeen years, the inexpressible weariness in her eyes, the fear that I would not be able to hold out and be here for her at the end if this wore on and on, all came together for me in one prayer, a cry from the heart spoken aloud as I finished the hymn.

"Lord, if it is your will, release her right now."

On the word now, like snapping a light switch from on to off, it happened. After twenty hours of waiting, wondering if each moment would be the last, wondering if it had already happened and I had missed it, I knew the very second of death. I felt her spirit brush by in passing, and she was gone.

Gone for now. I had no doubt to where she had gone, and I knew that I would meet her there again someday.

I checked my watch: 4:15. Mom's illness was over. The tears came as I stood there by the bed, and just a minute or so later, the aide came in with a fresh sheet under her arm. "I think she's gone," I managed, and she put down the sheet and turned away, saying, "I'll get my nurse."

It was the aide, not the nurse, who returned a few minutes later. She gave me a sympathetic rub across the back as she stepped around and studied Mom herself, reaching out to touch her face, cracking an eyelid to gently touch the eye. "Yes," she confirmed. She hit the bed controls, lowering the head of the bed. "No more pain," she said. "No more suffering."

"Yes. Singing in the heavenly choir now."

She picked up the stuffed tiger from the bed and handed it to me, then fingered the cat nightgown. "Do you want this? They'll just cut it off at the funeral home."

Cut it *off*? Such a cute cat nightgown? "Yes," I said. She went away for a hospital gown, then came back and changed Mom, handing the gown over to me. At that moment, a text arrived from Rena. Bless Rena. She and Dad were already up and thinking of me, even this early. The text was a promise, not a question, saying that they would be here between 8:00 and 9:00. I sent back a reply that it was all over, and then, one by one, I notified my three brothers and her sister.

Finally, the nurse arrived from whatever other patient she had been attending to. She pulled out her stethoscope, listened, listened again, moving it all over the chest, then stepped back and nodded.

"Do you want a few minutes alone with her before I start preparing her?" the aide asked.

"Yes," I replied, and they both withdrew, closing the door discreetly.

I sat down, the same position I'd had most of the night, but everything had changed. I ran one hand along her silver hair, and the only two words that came the whole time I sat there with her body were repeated again and again, telling her, telling Jesus. "Thank you. Thank you. Thank you."

Finally, I stood. I looked at her one last time, a pitiful, disease-wracked body. An empty body. She wasn't here anymore. Clutching the stuffed tiger and the cat nightgown, I left the room. The aide was in the common room, and another resident was there, already up. A new day was about to begin. "I'm leaving," I said. "Thank you all for everything."

She gave me another light touch on the arm. "I'm sorry. We loved your mother," she said.

I walked through the nursing home halls and out the front door. It was still dark, predawn, and as I left the facility, I stopped in surprise.

There, facing me at the end of the sidewalk up to the building, just where that pavement met the sidewalk that ran along next to the parking lot, sat a street cat. He was at attention, tail wrapped around, looking toward the doors as if he had come to pay final tribute to the patron saint of hungry, down-on-their-luck street cats. He looked as if he might have been carved in stone there. As I advanced down the sidewalk, he came to his feet, gave a leisurely feline stretch, and then walked off. It was a measured retreat; I had time to pull out my cell phone belatedly and snap a picture. I wished I had one of him sitting at attention wrapped in his tail at the end of the sidewalk at first, but at least I got the shot of him walking off.

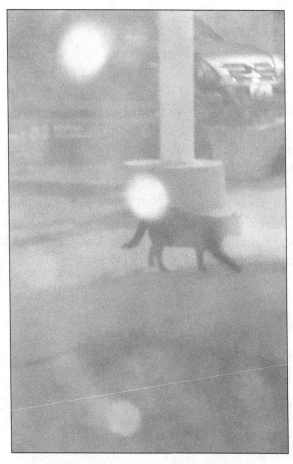

**"A street cat... come to pay final tribute."**

After he had left, I sat down in the car, then pulled up the picture and smiled. A street cat. How absolutely appropriate right then. No, I don't think it was Mom's spirit, but I do think that creation is more in tune at times with events than we realize, and I liked the thought that part of it was aware of something going on this night. God can speak through animals. God can speak even more through people, through family, and through a parent's love.

"Thank you," I said again.

Then I started the car and drove away. The nightmare of confusion was over. For Mom, the sunrise had come.

# 21.

# *Epilogue: No Appeal*

Nearly two months after her death, I wrote:

> *All sorts of things I encounter through the day remind me of her, and I love it. I love it because the things that remind me of her now are not bittersweet. Almost all of them remind me of her as she used to be, in her right mind, before the disease, and now, there is no downside of the second memory holding hard to the tail of the first that she is sick, that she isn't like that anymore. Now, she is free, and I can remember with unmixed feelings what she was like.*

Indeed, I found myself missing her less when she was dead than I did the final years of her life. I think most of the grieving truly was done while she was still alive, a living funeral that had seemed endless at times. Now, at last, that part was over.

I also felt her presence more. I could hear her voice, see her smile, share things with a mental nod that reminded me of her much more easily than I could during her illness. I had always had the memories; now, I had the release to go with them. She wasn't suffering anymore. I often imagined her enthusiasm up in heaven's choir.

And the laughter. Plenty of times, there was the laughter, like being able to share a joke with her once again.

A letter came from the state in September that was addressed to Mom and proudly proclaimed itself on the envelope to be "official business." I retrieved it from the mailbox as I turned into the farm driveway, and after driving on to my parking spot beside the house, I opened it there in the car, curious. What sort of official business could there be left? Had they, in fact, sent that prodigious form for her annual review as they had every autumn for many years? If so, I would enjoy sending it back for once without filling out each painstaking square.

No, this wasn't the annual review form. Instead, it informed Mom that her nursing home benefits had been cancelled for the following reason: death. They had conducted a search and couldn't find any substitute benefits for which she might be eligible. Mom had ninety days to appeal this decision; please see appeals process below.

I read that in disbelief, then burst into laughter right there in the car, watched by curious cats through the windshield. I could almost hear Mom laughing with me, could remember her voice saying as it had many times through the years, "Government efficiency is an oxymoron."

I was tempted briefly to file an appeal just to see the look on their faces at the hearing, but I decided against it. No, nothing would change their procedures or forms anyway. Bureaucracy was merely a lizard, not a dragon, and I had far better things to do with my time than suit up in armor and tackle it.

So now did Mom.

There would be no appeal. No benefits program the state could ever put together could match what Mom was living now.

I got out of the car, stroked the cats, and went on inside, depositing the letter in the trash can.

# *Credits*

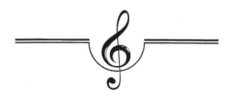

**Chapter 2** – Slaying Lizards

[1] Johnston, Julia H (1849-1919), "Grace Greater Than All Our Sin." Public domain. Quoted from https://hymnary.org/text/marvelous_grace_of_our_loving_lord

[2] Ephesians 4:32, *Holy Bible, King James Version.* Cambridge Edition: 1769.

[3] First Corinthians 14:40, *KJV.*

[4] Proverbs 12:10, *KJV.*

[5] Shakespeare, William (1564-1616), *Hamlet.* Act I, scene 5, line 109. Public domain. Quoted from https://www.goodreads.com/work/quotes/1885548-the-tragicall-historie-of-hamlet-prince-of-denmark

[6] Tilton, Theodore (1835-1907), "Even This Shall Pass Away." Public domain. Quoted from http://www.paulreapoetry.com/?p=626

## Chapter 3 – Partners

[7]Lazarus, Emma (1849-1887), "The New Colossus." Public domain. Quoted from https://www.poetryfoundation.org/poems/46550/the-new-colossus with one word modified as a family joke to fit Mom's cat-appeal.

[8] Second Corinthians 5:1, *KJV*.

## Chapter 4 – "If I Forget."

[9]Watts, Isaac (1674-1748), "Marching to Zion." Public domain. Quoted from https://hymnary.org/text/come_we_that_love_the_lord_and_let_our with words modified by Mom.

[10] Revelation 21:4, *KJV*.

[11] Philippians 1:3, *New American Standard Bible*. 1995. LaHabra, CA: The Lockman Foundation.

[12] Browning, Elizabeth Barrett (1806-1861), "Sonnet 43." Public domain. Quoted from https://www.poets.org/poetsorg/poem/how-do-i-love-thee-sonnet-43

[13] Browning, Robert (1812-1889), *Paracelsus*. Public domain. Quoted from "God, Thou Art Love" (Columbus: Beckenhorst Press, 2003).

[14] Newman, John Henry (1801-1890), "Lead, Kindly Light." Public domain. Quoted from https://hymnary.org/text/lead_kindly_light_amid_the_encircling_gl

**Chapter 5** – Moving to Erdenheim

[15] Psalm 23:6, *KJV.*

**Chapter 6** – Twilight

[16] Burns, Robert (1759-1796), "To a Mouse." Public domain. Quoted from https://www.poetryfoundation. org/poems/43816/to-a-mouse-56d222ab36e33

**Chapter 7** – Powerless.

[17] Washburn, Henry S. (1832-1871), "The Vacant Chair." Public domain. Quoted from https://allpoetry.com/ The-Vacant-Chair

**Chapter 8** – The Bad Summer

[18] Lathbury, Mary A. (1841-1913), "Day Is Dying in the West." Public domain. Quoted from https://www. hymnal.net/en/hymn/h/616

**Chapter 12** – Transfer

[19] Proverbs 25:11, *KJV.*

**Chapter 13** – The Roller Coaster

[20] Coleridge, Samuel Taylor (1772-1834), "Rime of the Ancient Mariner." Public domain. Quoted from https://www.poetryfoundation.org/poems/43997/ the-rime-of-the-ancient-mariner-text-of-1834

[21] Revelation 22:20, *KJV.*

**Chapter 14** – Diamonds

[22] Crosby, Frances (1820-1915), "Blessed Assurance." Public domain. Quoted from https://hymnary.org/text/blessed_assurance_jesus_is_mine

CPSIA information can be obtained
at www.ICGtesting.com
Printed in the USA
FFHW02n1019190918
48434972-52290FF